The Management of Voice Disorders

The Management of Voice Disorders

Murray Morrison

Head Division of Otolaryngology
The University of British Columbia
and Vancouver General Hospital
Canada

and

Linda Rammage

Speech Pathology Consultant and Research Director
Vancouver Voice Clinic
The University of British Columbia
Canada

with:

Hamish Nichol, *Psychiatrist*

Bruce Pullan, *Singing teacher*

Phillip May, *Singing teacher*

Lesley Salkeld, *Pediatric otolaryngologist*

Members of the Voice Clinic Team, Vancouver, British Columbia, Canada

SINGULAR PUBLISHING GROUP, INC.
San Diego, California

Singular Publishing Group, Inc.
4284 41st Street
San Diego, California 92105

First edition 1994

Typeset in 10/12 Palatino by Cotswold Typesetting Ltd, Gloucester

Printed in Great Britain by TJ Press (Padstow) Ltd, Cornwall

ISBN 1 56593 311 7

A catalogue record for this book is available from the British Library

Library of Congress Cataloging-in-Publication data available

"... to our families ..."

Contents

Preface

There has been a tremendous growth of interest in the human voice and its disorders during the past decade. This has led to the development of a variety of 'voice labs' or 'voice clinics' that are able to offer unique interdisciplinary assessment and treatment facilities. To cover all the bases, the voice care team requires input from laryngology, speech-language pathology, psychiatry, neurology, voice science, music pedagogy, biomedical engineering and other peripheral fields. Because of the multidisciplinary nature of voice clinics there have been a number of books written that address our subject from different professional perspectives. These tend to be multi-authored works that draw on expertise from around the world, such as a laryngologist from New York, a speech pathologist from Toronto, etc. All are colleagues that share similar interests but never actually share the management problems of the same patients.

This book has been planned and written by the members of a single 'voice clinic'. It is our hope that it will reflect a singleness of direction and purpose in the way it presents our approach to a complex topic. Because of our regular interactive meetings over problem patients in which we debate the meaning of our observations, the evolution of etiological classification systems, and the rationale for particular therapy approaches, we feel that we have become a team that is greater than the sum of its parts, and that there is value in sharing our cumulative thoughts with others.

This is not simply a laryngology text for laryngologists. Neither is it a speech pathology text exclusively for speech pathologists . . . we hope that this text will fill in the gaps between the professions that must work together for the benefit of the voice disordered patient. It should expand the understanding of medical and surgical laryngology for the singing teacher, and should help to demystify the art of vocal pedagogy for both the laryngologist and the speech pathologist. It should help the psychiatrist appreciate the ways in which muscle misuses lead to dysphonia, and provide some extra tools to the speech pathologist embarking on a therapy program with a psychologically unbalanced patient.

Our clinic is the product of who we are, where we live, the politics of our health care system, where and how we were educated, the expectations of our clientele, and an assortment of personal biases. No other clinic group can be the same or share just the same philosophies. Some will function more effectively and some less so. Should you be heading in a similar direction we hope that you too will find that learning from each other is fun and rewarding.

Murray Morrison
Linda Rammage

Acknowledgements

The many original and redrawn illustrations in this book have been done by Frank Crymble, Bambi Edlund and Jane Rowlands. Dr Joseph Tsui provided helpful advice on the neurological aspects of the manuscript and Susan Kernested provided extensive secretarial assistance. The authors extend thanks to these individuals.

1

Evaluation of the voice-disordered patient

The information in this and subsequent chapters assumes familiarity with basic anatomy and current theories of physiology of the speech and voice mechanism. The reader who is not in possession of this knowledge base is encouraged to begin by reading Chapter 10 in this text, supplemented with additional recommended readings.

1.1 PRINCIPLES OF JOINT ASSESSMENT

It is usual in medical practice to evaluate a constellation of signs and symptoms, and from them to deduce a diagnosis. Once the diagnosis has been secured, treatment is planned. Voice disorders tend to be managed differently, at least those with a spectrum of causes. A successful treatment program must address all of the causative factors. For example, a mild habitual technical voice misuse may be exacerbated by psychological factors, while the smooth operation of the pharyngolaryngo-esophageal muscular tube is inhibited by mild gastric reflux, and the disordered voice is finally triggered by an acute viral infection. The viral trigger will spontaneously disappear but the other three factors need separate attention and, since a fully successful result will require coordinated medical treatment, voice therapy, and psychological support, we find that the voice-disordered person gets help most efficiently from a multidisciplinary team.

'What one knows one sees'. There is no substitute for an informed and aware clinician in the evaluation of a voice-disordered patient. On the other hand, complete objectivity is a rare achievement for a clinician working alone. Interdisciplinary evaluation offers the best chance of identifying all aspects of pathogenesis contributing to voice disorders.

One day after the initial interview with a 44-year-old aphonic patient, conducted by the laryngologist, speech pathologist and psychiatrist, the first comment in the ensuing conference was from the psychiatrist: 'What an incredible amount of anger is being suppressed by this lady!' She had been whispering for over a year and exhibited the type of symptom inconsistencies that would lead an informed clinician to suspect a psychogenic etiology: normal cough and laughter were observed although she was aphonic during speech; and incomplete glottic closure was noted during a sustained /i/ on indirect laryngoscopy although complete closure was demonstrated during a spontaneous cough and inhalation phonation. To the untrained or biased eye or ear, however, the key etiological factors could have been easily missed.

The team evaluation provides a multiple-observer situation. While the otolaryngologist or speech pathologist is conducting the interview, the other team member(s) are free to make general observations that might be missed by the interviewer, particularly if he or she were conducting the interview alone. Further, by joining forces, team members bring different areas of expertise into the evaluation process, while diluting each others' reductive biases.

Incidentally, the lady mentioned above spent a couple of hours, mostly in tears, with the psychiatrist, and normal speech was restored during voice therapy the following day. Due to an ongoing difficult social situation, it is likely that the aphonia will be resumed because of the protective role it plays in her life.

In our clinic we solicit information in advance of the voice evaluation, from those making patient referrals. It is obviously not economical or sensible to involve a psychiatrist or psychologist with every voice patient, much less at the initial interview. Reports from the referring consultants may give clues to major psychological components, which enables us to schedule such patients for evaluation at times when the psychiatrist is present. In most cases difficult barriers are broken down by this interdisciplinary introduction, saving valuable therapy time.

Owing to time and economic constraints, it may not be possible to have the speech pathologist attend each patient evaluation. A review of the referral letters will often identify those patients that have a strictly organic laryngeal disorder requiring only the services of the laryngologist initially. In our experience, for the majority of cases it seems advisable to have the otolaryngologist and speech pathologist see patients together from the outset, each bringing their own professional skills to the evaluation process. This way, the two professionals can contribute to a common data base for patient management, and perhaps most importantly, they can provide a comprehensive assessment service, while learning from each other's skills. By employing team assessment strategies consistently, professionals reach a deeper understanding of the nature of the complexities manifesting themselves in voice-disordered patients.

To summarize the principles alluded to above, it is important to secure detailed referral information so as to be able to decide which professionals to have at the first interview. Joint assessment is obviously time-consuming and at first, may not appear to be cost-efficient. To the contrary, a well-orchestrated, interdisciplinary assessment strategy provides a forum for shared observations based on multiobserver perceptions, and is the most efficient way to reach immediate consensus about treatment priorities and plans.

1.2 HISTORY TAKING

1.2.1 Rationale and Philosophy

Taking the history from a voice-disordered patient can be a complex and time-consuming process. Consequently it does not readily fit into the usual patient flow of a typical medical practice. In a multidisciplinary voice clinic, the initial history taking may be performed by various individuals including a laryngologist, speech pathologist, resident, or speech pathology intern. With one primary historytaker designated to a patient, other team members present can make and record observations of behavior that are helpful in arriving at the diagnosis. Time constraints in a busy medical practice can make this process a luxury. In such situations the laryngologist or speech pathologist may conduct the initial interview alone with the patient, followed by any clinical and instrumental assessment activities reflecting the expertise of that clinician's discipline. The other team members see the patient subsequent to this, and may review and amplify the history, then proceed with their own assessment procedures. The principal diagnostic opinion will be formed by the primary history taker and others who are in attendance at the initial interview, since it is this process that provides the most useful information.

Figure 1.1 illustrates the 'history' part of the printed form that we use in our clinic. It facilitates an orderly movement through the process regardless of who conducts the interview. The format serves as a quality assurance tool, by ensuring that each relevant topic is presented and reported in the history. A brief comment will be made about each section. It is important to come to an agreement about the nature of questions asked during the interview. Consistent with principles of objective history taking, each interviewer practices use of open-ended questions during the primary interview. This strategy guards against simple 'yes/no' responses to specific leading questions that may bias the clinician toward a particular diagnosis before all the facts are available. Ideally, the interviewer's questions guide a patient to disclose specific information without leading him or her to respond in a clinician-biased manner so as to 'fit' a diagnostic model. Examples of open-ended phrases employed to direct the discussion include:

- 'Tell me all you can about how your speech or throat are troubling you.';
- 'Tell me about any patterns you may have noticed in these symptoms.';
- 'Tell me about your job/family/childhood/hobbies.';
- 'Tell me about any other illnesses or health concerns.';
- 'Describe a typical day/week in your life.'.

1.2.2 Chronology of the Problem as it Unfolded

This text cannot cover the entire art of taking a basic history but a few points are worth making. Of greatest importance is the recognition that a multiplicity of etiological factors may contribute to symptom formation.

Organic disease can trigger a muscle misuse dysphonia, so that what appears initially to be a straightforward viral laryngitis may evolve into a long-lasting voice disorder.

VGH Voice Clinic   4th Floor Willow Pavilion,   Vancouver General Hospital 875-4204

NAME: AGE: SEX: DATE:

Chief Complaint: Duration:

History:

Occupation: _____

Type of voice use_____

Voice training_____

Past Medical History:

Allergies _____
Diet/weight: _____
Smoking (1°/2°) _____
Alcohol _____
Coffee/tea_____
Reflux:
   • globus _____
   • p.n. drip_____
   • throat clearing _____
   • heart burn _____
   • am throat _____
   • acid taste _____
   • water brash_____
   • night chokes_____
Reflux diagnosis? (Y/N)_____
Hearing _____
Audiogram? (Y/N) _____

VOCAL ABUSE HISTORY	Severity/Observations
Throat clearing/coughing	
Shouting/cheering/(+ emotive)	
Screaming/yelling/crying (−)	
Talking over noise (specify)	
Talking outdoors/pools etc.	
Lecturing, etc. (poor amplif)	
Voice use & strenuous exercise	
Non verbal vocal sounds	
Imitating voices	
Stage whisper	
Excessive singing, talking, etc	
Other: (specify)	

FAMILY HISTORY

PSYCHOLOGICAL/STRESS FACTORS

PATIENTS PERCEPTION OF VOICE DISORDER

Severity/Variability _____

Impact/expectation_____

Singer? (Y/N) _____ Status:_____ Range: S A T B

Singers Questionaire filled out? (Y/N) _____

Figure 1.1 Form for history taking.

Koufman and Blalock refer to this as 'habituated hoarseness' [31]. In this situation a subclinical voice misuse may be brought to the surface when coupled with inflammatory edema, and then persist when the edema subsides. Muscle misuse and vocal abuse disorders tend to worsen as the day, week, or duration of use proceeds, but may also fluctuate with stresses of other sorts described below. An open, puzzle-solving frame of mind will help the history taker receive such clues and hypothesize on the significance of reported symptom patterns.

1.2.3 Family History

Voice disorders, particularly those that are psychologically based, may be associated with relationships that are first glimpsed during discussion about family members. Talking about the family is a good way to get to know a patient, and also provides information about familial patterns of speech and voice problems, such as are common with benign essential tremor.

1.2.4 Psychological Factors and Stressors

Dysphonias of psychological etiology tend to occur in persons who are restraining the impulse to cry or in those who are suppressing anger. Although these behaviors are often detectable through nonverbal clues, it may be necessary to ask some direct questions to open doors to potentially important areas. Critical events such as childhood sexual abuse or other past violence may be so deeply buried that they will not emerge during the voice assessment except perhaps in session with the psychiatrist. Of course, these events may or may not play a significant role in symptom formation of the current voice problem. To obtain straightforward information about how patients respond to stressful situations it is often helpful to ask them to rate themselves on a scale of 1 to 10, with one representing a very relaxed person and 10 representing anxious or 'uptight'. The response is followed by a request to describe situations that contribute to stress. We are interested in knowing the social context in which the dysphonia was first manifested, what anxiety-laden thoughts the patient was seeking to deal with, what other emotions were aroused at the time, and whether these were suppressed or overtly expressed. As the patient recounts these events, the history taker notes changes in body posture indicative of tension, especially those related to alterations in voice production. More detail about the psychological relationships associated with voice disorders is covered in section 1.3 and Chapter 5.

1.2.5 Patient's Perception of the Voice Disorder

We are interested in finding out what impact the voice disorder has had on a patient, by means of open-ended probing. It is surprising how often a patient seems devastated about something that to the clinician appears trivial, and vice versa. The impact may relate to changes or restrictions in occupational, social, or psychological dimensions.

1.2.6 Medical History and Reflux

Health, allergies, smoking, diet, alcohol, etc. are all important but the question of possible underlying reflux esophagitis needs special attention. If one probes about globus, postnasal drip, habitual throat clearing, sour acid taste and heartburn; and whether these are worse first thing in the morning, or whether the patient wakes at night choking, coughing, or wheezing, then a fairly clear picture of the presence or absence of significant reflux will emerge. It is tempting to generate specific leading questions when probing for reflux symptomatology, since the information being sought is specific. As with all history areas, it is critical to present this topic as objectively as possible, so as not to lead patients to hasty 'yes/no' responses to diagnostic terms that may not adequately describe their symptoms, thus resulting in misdiagnosis.

There are often a number of factors involved in the genesis of a voice disorder, unlike some other medical conditions where a number of signs and symptoms relate to diagnosis of a single illness. For example, a postural or habitual technical voice misuse may set the stage, an emotionally trying social situation provides the script, reflux produces a jumpy irritable laryngo-esophageal neuromuscular system, and a viral infection opens the curtain.

Hearing acuity must be considered, both that of the patient and of his or her communication partners. Presbycusis in an elderly person reduces the ability to adequately monitor his or her own voice, and vocal fold atrophy or degeneration may compound the communication disability. Consider also the compounding effect of a voice-disordered individual with a hearing-impaired spouse or parent when judging the severity or impact of dysphonia.

1.2.7 Vocal Abuse History

Some information on vocal abuses may have been covered during general questioning, but it is useful to review the specific abusive behaviors and their severity. Look and listen for clues to the following:

- throat clearing and habitual coughing;
- positive emotional abuse such as cheering;
- negative emotional overuse such as crying or screaming;
- talking over noise or in poor acoustic environments;
- lecturing or singing with poor amplification;
- voice use with strenuous exercise;
- nonverbal vocal sounds;
- imitating voices or stage whisper;
- excessive singing, talking, yelling.

1.3 PSYCHOLOGICAL EVALUATION

When the psychological examination of a patient is conducted jointly with the laryngologist and speech pathologist, the role of the psychiatrist is immediately made clear to the patient: the psychiatrist is an individual with particular interests in, and expertise about psychological factors that may cause the dysphonia, or those which arise in consequence of having a poor voice. It helps in establishing rapport if the psychiatrist is not viewed as someone looking for signs of insanity. It is valuable for the psychiatrist to observe the changes in a patient's voice, emotional status and posture that may occur while the laryngologist or speech pathologist is taking the initial history. During the joint interview, the psychiatrist may interject to elicit additional information specific to the patient's psychological status. As a physician trained to ensure that an underlying physical condition has not been overlooked before one plunges into the psychological realm, it is reassuring to the psychiatrist to have had the opportunity to view a videotaped image of the laryngoscopy examination.

The laryngologist uses the videotape to explain the significance of the findings to the patient, who then knows that the psychiatrist is aware of any lesions or lack thereof, or any muscle misuses contributing to dysphonia. Where the larynx is demonstrated to be free of organic disorders but is being misused, the stage is set for review of other factors: social, psychological, and emotional.

After the laryngoscopy and phonatory function measures have been completed by the other team members, an individual interview by the psychiatrist is indicated. It has been our finding that patients are more forthcoming in describing personal problems in this situation. It is useful to begin the interview by reassuring patients that the idea their dysphonia is 'all in their heads' is nonsense. By producing a dysphonic voice himself, the psychiatrist demonstrates that misuse of the muscles of phonation are responsible for the dysphonic voice. It is explained that while this is being created deliberately by the clinician, the patient's dysphonia arises from some habitual misuse outside of his or her awareness, the causes of which now need to be sought. Dependent on a patient's history, examples are offered of dysphonia resulting from the operation of infection, reflux, or overuse, coupled with a stressful social situation which did not permit the overt expression of the emotions raised by the distressing ideas.

Another example of a common psychological mechanism in symptom formation is apprehension and physical tension produced by the anticipation of a dysphonic voice when answering the telephone. With this type of introduction, some increase in rapport has usually been achieved and patients are generally receptive to the idea of looking for the factors that could have produced the dysphonia. This is especially the case when there is the mutual awareness that no structural abnormalities were found on laryngoscopy, or that those identified could not account fully for the dysphonia. In those instances where the psychiatrist was not present for the initial evaluation, it is advisable to review the videotape of the laryngoscopy and any diagnostic therapy, to inform the patient that this has been done, and to establish with the patient a mutual understanding of what had been demonstrated.

Review of the history of the dysphonia as given to the laryngologist or speech pathologist is then undertaken with particular emphasis on the patient's life situation at the start of each episode of dysphonia. In doing so, close observation is made of any changes in the patient's voice related to specific topics, especially those of emotionally charged situations or significant relationships. Dependent upon circumstances, it may or may not be desirable to draw a patient's attention to decreases or increases in the dysphonia and to relate this to the subject being discussed. Usually it is wise to wait until there have been two or three significant changes in voice before making the patient aware of the connection. At this point, asking how the patient accounts for the changes will often lead to much more declarative statements being made about significant psychological factors. It is worthwhile pursuing any events that have impinged on the neck area, such as a thyroidectomy, being choked in a fight, or a whiplash injury resulting from a car accident, which may have occurred prior to any report of dysphonia. A patient will often say that his or her neck has long been a vulnerable area. In addition, it is useful to determine how the patient experiences stress. Dysphonic patients commonly report headaches, shoulder tension, or breathing difficulties.

The usual psychiatric history is obtained with emphasis on how the expression of emotionally charged ideas were accepted in the family of origin, and later in adult life, at work, or in the family of procreation. The determination of a patient's self-percept is important. Does the patient perceive him or herself to be passive, unsuccessful and mild in manner and voice; or domineering, declarative and loudly successful, with no idea of how a dysphonia could possibly have arisen? Individuals falling into the latter group, it should be noted, are rather unlikely to be willing to accept the operation of psychological factors in their voice disorders. How much is the patient's voice a valued, central part of his or her central identity? As D.H. Lawrence [34] has written in his poem 'The Oxford Voice':

When you hear it languishing
and hooing and cooing and sidling through the front teeth
the Oxford voice
or worse still
the would-be Oxford voice
you don't even laugh any more, you can't . . .
We wouldn't insist on it for a moment
but we are
we are
you admit we are
superior.

For a professional voice user or an amateur poseur, any dysphonia strikes close to home. Voices that are indicative of significant personality traits and coping styles invariably require a peculiar use of the muscles of phonation to produce them. It is not a patient's 'natural voice' if it is whining, sycophantic, bombastic, or shrill. It is, then, particularly important to determine how patients' premorbid personalities enable them to respond to the advent of the psychiatric disorder, such as a depressive illness, post-traumatic stress disorder, adjustment reaction, or anxiety disorder, to mention the commonest ones we encounter, and how the voice becomes embroiled in an individual's response.

In conducting the direct mental status examination, attention should be paid to the attitude and general behavior of the patient, particularly with regard to voice production. To what extent is a patient's preoccupation with dysphonia at variance with the degree of the disability? It is important to note the patient's affective responses, especially those of anxiety, anger, and sadness, whether covert or overt. These emotions, if not expressed freely without conflict are particularly likely to have an impact on phonation. Nonverbal cues, such as changes in facial expression or alterations in posture when the patient is talking about certain topics, are often revealing, particularly when they are accompanied by changes in the quality, pitch or loudness of the patient's voice. A worsening of dysphonia may be noted when certain subjects are discussed. Engaging the patient in a lively, affectively charged conversation, thus causing a distraction from the dysphonia, at times leads to a significant improvement in voice, a fact that has diagnostic significance.

Having completed the full psychiatric examination, including, where indicated, a detailed mental status examination, it is often useful to request the patient's permission to examine them for evidence of physical tension. The laryngologist and speech pathologist will already have examined the larynx and articulators. Palpating the short rotators of the head and evaluating the movement of the head on the neck, the freedom of neck and shoulder movements, as well as how the patient's respiration changes while this is being done, provides useful supplementary information. It is not common to misuse the intrinsic muscles of phonation without having an inappropriate level of tension in the auxiliary muscles of the head, neck, chest, and abdomen. After all, the larynx is suspended between the jaw, neck, and upper chest; if the intrinsic muscles are very tense, the auxiliary muscles usually are too, hence the common postural abnormalities observed in dysphonic patients. It is useful to observe the patient's respiration, particularly a tendency to increase intra-abdominal pressure in order to be able to force air through constricted vocal folds. Drawing patients' attention to tightness of the abdominal wall, spasm of the pelvic floor and rigidity of the chest gives them a much better idea of why they produce peculiar vocal sounds, especially when they are emotionally aroused but not willing to express their feelings fully.

Dependent on the degree of psychological factors producing the dysphonia and the receptivity of the patient to the idea that these are in operation, comments are made promptly to the patient. In those instances where there are a multiplicity of factors operating, or the patient has a distinct desire for an organic explanation for the dysphonia, little is said. Rather, the need for a conference with the laryngologist and speech pathologist is emphasized. In such cases, it is important that the laryngologist and speech pathologist provide the summary statement and be the ones to direct the treatment plan, whether it involves primary voice therapy or concurrent psychological treatment with medical procedures or voice rehabilitation. It is often useful for all three professionals to be together with the patient when this is done.

1.4 ACOUSTIC AND PERCEPTUAL-ACOUSTIC ASSESSMENT

1.4.1 Rationale, Environment and Basic Recording Hardware

Perceptual assessment methods, both visual and auditory, provide valuable information during assessment of voice-disordered patients. Techniques for assessing anatomical and vibratory features of the phonatory mechanism will be discussed in a subsequent section. Perceptual-acoustic evaluation provides the critical information link between physiological voice function and a listener's perception of the resultant acoustic speech signal. Since the listener's auditory system filters and processes the radiated acoustic speech signal before it is interpreted by the brain, perceptual-acoustic evaluation provides a uniquely 'human' set of information regarding voice function or dysfunction, for example the appropriateness of speaking pitch, loudness, and voice quality.

High quality acoustic recordings are essential for reliable perceptual and digital acoustic evaluation. A sound-treated recording studio is recommended in cases where the evaluation room is not sound-proofed, or contains noise-generating equipment that must be kept running during the acoustic recording. Audio and video recordings of vocal status before and after intervention are necessary to document treatment efficacy. Simultaneous video recording allows the observation of concurrent posture, movement, and acoustic aspects of voice production. Both clinician and patient benefit from documentation, and the medicolegal value of high-quality recordings has proven itself on several occasions. Cassette recorders allow for easy and efficient storage and retrieval of patient data. Digital recording devices are ideal for acoustic recordings that will be subjected to further acoustic analysis, owing to their superior quality, and they avoid the need for analog-to-digital processing. A unidirectional microphone is generally better than an omnidirectional microphone for realistic recordings, especially where background noise is not well controlled. The microphone needs to have good feedback suppression, a low distortion factor, and a wide frequency range representing the typical spectrum for speech sounds, and any atypical speech and voice noise that may characterize dysphonias. An ideal frequency response ranges from near O Hz, to 20 KHz.

1.4.2 Acoustic Assessment: Instrumentation, Application, Protocols and Interpretation

High quality acoustic recordings, either analog or digital, should be made as a standard assessment procedure for each voice patient, regardless of etiology or treatment plan. The comprehensive acoustic evaluation includes assessment of pitch, loudness, rate/duration, and quality parameters of phonation and speech. The form in Figure 1.2 is used to guide the speech pathologist through assessment tasks, and to record findings. Assessment tasks are designed to elicit 'typical' and maximal voice range data, and include speech and nonspeech contexts. Ideally, candid recordings of speech and/or performance in typical voice-use situations are used to assess the range of phonatory behaviors and difficulties experienced by a patient.

Fundamental Frequency/Pitch and Intensity/Loudness

In the clinic, instrumental measures can be used to define speech averages, and dynamic ranges for fundamental frequency (f_0) and intensity of phonation. Average speaking f_0 and range are extracted from contextual speech, while physiological range for f_0 is

PERCEPTUAL-ACOUSTIC FEATURES

PITCH PARAMETERS

Singing Range: High:_____ (asc.); _____ (desc.)Register:_____

(Hz/Note)   Low: _____ (asc.): _____ (desc.)Register:_____

Total range: _____ Flexibility/continuity: _____

Register transisitions:_____ (asc.):_____ (desc.)

Speaking Range: High:_____ Low:_____ Habitual:_____
(average)

(Hz)   Situational variability:_____ Intonation:_____

/o of non verbal vocal sounds: um hm/uh huh: _____

hm/huh: _____ laugh: _____ cough/thr. clear: _____

Appropriateness of speaking pitch, range, register: _____

Pitch-matching: _____ Musicality:_____

LOUDNESS PARAMETERS

SPL Range: High: a < _____ ; serials < _____ ; "Hey" _____

Low: a > _____ ; serials > _____ ; "Hey" _____

Habitual (average) SPL Level-Speech: _____ Situational Variability: _____

Cough strength: _____ Pitch/Loudness Interdependence _____

RATE/DURATION PARAMETERS:

Sustained Phonemes: a _____ , _____ , _____ m_____ , _____

(duration/sec.)   max.: _____ Cued? (Y/N) _____

s/z ratio: _____

Connected Speech: Serials max. duration:_____ (rate+3 digits/sec.)

Habitual (average) Rate of Speech: _____ Average Phrase Length:_____

Fluency: _____ Fluency/Rate Variability:_____

QUALITY PARAMETERS:

	0	1 2	3 4 5	6 7
	N	Mild	Moderate	Severe

Voice-Onset Features:	Sev. Freq.	Consistency/Stimulability	Valving Features:	Sev. Freq	Consistency/Stimulability
Glottal Attack			Breathy		
Hyperadd-Delayed Onset			Whisper phonation-unforced		
Hypoadd-Delayed Onset			Stage Whisper forced		
Hyperadducted Release			Hypervalved (squeezed)		
Breath-Intake Features:			Timbre/Dissonance Features:		
Inspiratory Stridor-laryngeal			Strident/Harsh (♪pitch)		
Audible Inspiration-unvoiced			Rough/Glottal Fry (♪ pitch)		
Inhalation phonation/speech			Diplophonic/Glottal Fry		
Stability Features:			Resonance Features:		
Tremolo			Hypernasality/consonant emission		
Tremor			Assimilative nasality-vowels		
Pitch Breaks (specify♪♪)			Hyponasality (m. n, ng)		
Hyperadd Phonation Breaks			Fronted Resonance/Artic		
Hypoadd Phonation Breaks			Backed Resonance		

STIMULABILITY FOR CHANGE IN PITCH, LOUDNESS, RATE, QUALITY PARAMETERS: _____

_____

_____

_____

_____

_____

_____

Figure 1.2 Form for acoustic and perceptual-acoustic assessment.

measured from singing scales and glissando productions. The same contextual speech sample may be used to measure average vocal intensity and range, whereas 'quietest' and 'loudest' productions are elicited on a simple word: *Hey!* or phrase: *Hey you!* Many dedicated instruments and software programs are now available to allow for such measures to be made accurately and efficiently in the voice clinic. Tried-and-true basic sound measurement devices such as the oscilloscope (for f_0 measurement) and the sound-level meter (for intensity measurement) are still valuable instruments for these physical measures. Electroglottography (EGG) can be used for accurate estimates of f_0 provided the voice is not too noisy.

The **phonetogram** provides a clinically relevant display of physiological ranges for f_0 and intensity and their interactions [12, 21, 30, 39]. Several software programs have been developed to measure and plot intensity range against f_0 range on a simple $x-y$ scale (Figure 1.3). This allows the patient and clinician to measure and compare changes in vocal dynamics over time. The phonetogram has enjoyed particular popularity within the arena of vocal pedagogy, and has been used to document differences between trained and untrained singers [1, 2, 22].

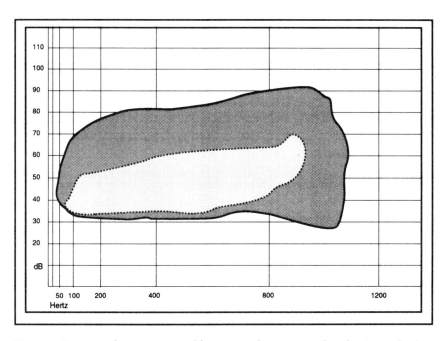

Figure 1.3 Prototype phonetogram: vocal frequency and intensity are plotted against each other to indicate ranges for each, and the relationship between these two acoustic variables. The x axis represents fundamental frequency; the y axis represents intensity of the vocal range. The phonetogram profiles for a patient pre- and post-treatment are demonstrated: the pretreatment plot is in light shading; the post-treatment in dark shading.

Although the physical parameters f_0 and acoustic intensity correspond closely to perceptual judgments of pitch and loudness respectively, the unique and complex nature of perceptual processing justifies clinical assessment of psychoacoustic parameters separately. Trained listeners have the unique ability to translate the physical signal to judgements regarding the 'appropriateness' of vocal pitch or loudness within a given communication context. The clinician can also determine the extent to which a speaker can use pitch and loudness changes effectively to produce natural suprasegmental characteristics of intonation and stress.

Normative data has been discrepant for physiological or artistic f_0 ranges, although generally a physiological pitch range of two octaves or greater is cited as the 'normal' critical range. A patient may have a greatly restricted physiological range (for example, less than one octave) and yet maintain a fully functional speaking voice with adequate intonation. On the other hand, a vocal performer with even subtle changes or restrictions in the dynamic range may suffer great occupational and emotional repercussions. Many vocal performers must produce aesthetically appropriate vocal tones that cover a range of three octaves.

The pitch range of an individual's speaking voice may be a problem if it draws undue attention to itself due to its variance from the socially accepted range of 'normal' for the age, sex, race, and linguistic code of the person. A speaking fundamental frequency range that is too low, too high or limited in its dynamics may result in psychosocial difficulties (or may in some cases serve to 'resolve' psychosocial conflicts). Speaking pitch ranges that are not representative of natural pitches produced on spontaneous phonation (eg. *um hum*; *uh huh*; laughing) usually are related to muscle misuse. These often lead to monotone speech, glottal fry, falsetto, or a high-pitched, tense voice. If an individual's inappropriate speaking pitch reflects the same range as that produced during spontaneous vocalizations, it is usually related primarily to anatomical features. Mass-altering lesions, endocrine disease, neurological disease, or congenital malformations may all lead to abnormally high, low, or reduced speaking pitch ranges. Vocal tract length and shape, and articulatory style can also affect speaking pitch. Longer or larger vocal tracts tend to be associated with lower formant frequencies which complement phonation at lower fundamental frequencies in men to give the perception of lower pitch, and the converse is true for women and children. In the case of a mismatch between resonance tract size and vocal f_0, as with adolescents with transitional dysphonias or individuals undergoing gender reassignment, pitch perception may be confounded. If a male-to-female transsexual consciously shortens her vocal tract length by raising the larynx, she may overcome the f_0–resonance mismatch by raising formant frequencies. The 'feminine voice' perception may be further influenced by a fronted and exaggerated articulatory style, and adoption of feminine intonation characteristics, all of which appear to influence listeners impressions of a higher vocal pitch. If these characteristics are combined with a mean f_0 in the gender-ambiguous range (around 160 Hz), they may influence the listener's decision toward 'feminine' identity [52]. The issue of pitch and vocal identity may pose a problem for some individuals during senescence, since f_0 tends to rise in men, and lower in women as a normal aging characteristic. This problem is discussed further in Chapter 8.

A monotone speaking style may reflect personality or psychological features: schizophrenia and affective disorders such as depression have been associated with reduced intonation patterns [14]. Muscle misuse in the larynx and supraglottic musculature may also lead to reduced vocal flexibility and monotone speech patterns. Neurogenic disease affecting the upper or lower motor neurons may also affect f_0 and pitch control. Lesions of the recurrent or superior laryngeal nerve may result in restricted pitch range, due to impaired vocal fold adduction and cricothyroid muscle dysfunction. Whereas a restricted speaking pitch range may be a consequence of a variety of psychological, muscle misuse and organic etiologies, abnormally wide speaking pitch ranges are seen only rarely, but might be expected in cases of certain psychological states, personality disorders or organic brain syndromes such as Gilles de la Tourette's syndrome.

Normative studies of maximum and minimum intensities for different age and sex groups suggest that a minimum dynamic (physiological) intensity range of approximately 30 dB or greater indicates normal voice function for adults [6, 24]. It is clear that the f_0 of phonation influences maximum and minimum intensity values, as does age to a lesser degree (see Baken [4] for a thorough review of data). Restrictions on the upper or lower end of the range may pose situation-specific problems for an individual. A reduced dynamic intensity range or inappropriate habitual loudness may be indicative of organic or muscle misuse disorders. Various peripheral and central neurological diseases may contribute to problems of vocal fold adduction (too much or too little) which affect ability to achieve the appropriate subglottic pressure for intensity increases or decreases. Respiratory diseases or incoordination may also contribute to intensity problems, if they impair one's ability to maintain sufficient air flow to create appropriate subglottic pressure. Finally, vocal intensity ranges may be affected by resonance characteristics. Structural or neurological disorders, and muscle misuse may result in acoustic damping due to poor oral opening, losses through the velopharyngeal port, or articulatory postures that affect the vocal tract transfer function. Inappropriate speaking intensity may be related to disease processes alluded to above, habitual misuse, hearing deficits, ambient noise levels, psychological conflict, or personality traits.

Rate and Duration

The rate of an individual's speech may affect coordination of respiration and phonation, muscular tension in the vocal tract, and intelligibility. Speaking rate may be influenced by situational, physiological, and personality factors. A well-trained speech clinician can generally make a perceptual judgement regarding the appropriateness of an individual's speaking rate for a given situation. Syllable or word counts for a series of typical speech utterances provide a more objective measure. A review of normative data suggests that the critical range for normal speaking rates may vary from 140 words per minute to 180 w.p.m. Of course the communication context, articulatory proficiency and other production variables must be considered when one is judging the appropriateness of speaking rate for a communication situation.

Measures of phonation duration include the traditional maximum phonation time (MPT) measure for sustained vowels at natural pitch and loudness within the speech range, as well as measures of speech phrase length. When interpreted in light of other phonatory function measures, MPT values can provide information regarding glottic integrity and/or respiratory support. The role of MPT in making phonation quotient calculations is discussed in section 1.5. Normative studies of MPT provide a wide variety of suggested guidelines for this measure. Age and sex variables are clearly both influential in determining normative ranges. For children, the average normative ranges reflect values from 13.1 s to 16.2 s, up to eight year of age. For adults, average values for females vary from 16.7 s to 25.7 s, and for males from 22 s to 34.6 s (see review by Hirano [24]).

Phrase lengths vary normally under the influence of syntax and pragmatics. A syllable or word count per phrase (expiratory breath group) can give the clinician objective data to supplement perceptual judgements of appropriateness of average phrase length. Phrase length may be influenced by rate of speech, with much longer average breath groups associated with rapid speech.

Perceptual or mathematical measures of phonatory fluency and rhythm may be included in the rate and duration evaluation. If syllable lengths are grossly variant owing to phonatory or articulatory dysfluency (for example, laryngeal or oral articulator blocks), then speech may be dysrhythmic or bizarre. Voice-onset delays due to hyper- or hypoadduction of the vocal folds may also disturb speech fluency and rhythm.

An excellent screening tool for identification of prosody and voice disorders has been developed by Shriberg, Kwiatkowski and Rasmussen [48]. The test battery provides a detailed training program, and scoring protocol for delineating phrasing, rate, and stress abnormalities, or voice abberations related to loudness, pitch, and quality that warrant more indepth evaluation.

Voice quality

Perceptual-acoustic terms employed to describe dysphonia features should reflect mechanical events that account for them. The terms for voice-quality measurement listed in our protocol for acoustic and perceptual-acoustic evaluation, are based on this philosophy (Figure 1.2). Laver's Vocal Profiles Analysis protocol [32, 33] employs similar principles for voice quality assessment and includes perceptual parameters corresponding to long-term postural settings within the phonatory, articulatory and resonance systems. Both these assessment protocols have been used in our clinic for detailed description of voice-quality features. Simultaneous acoustic, laryngoscopic, or EGG measures may be used to confirm the nature of phonatory events that correspond to perceptual judgements of pitch, loudness, rate-duration, and quality, and to train listeners to use perceptual terms reliably. Team members are trained to apply a common operational definition to each term, and high inter-listener reliability scores are sought for severity judgements. It is valuable to include a perceptual measure of social validation in the voice-assessment protocol. This may include use of bipolar, semantic differential scales (e.g. 'young'–'old'; 'steady'–'shaky') for non-professional evaluation [20]. By soliciting perceptual ratings from the public, the clinician and patient may gain a more realistic idea of the psychosocial impact a voice disorder has with respect to the 'average' listener during day-to-day discourse.

The voice quality assessment includes evaluation of upper vocal tract resonance characteristics. The primary evaluation technique used is perceptual-acoustic. Laver's Vocal Profile Analysis protocol is used to provide a comprehensive assessment of upper vocal tract postures [33]. Acoustic analysis techniques may provide additional information regarding formant frequencies, which reflect articulatory postures, or aspects of nasal resonance. The common neurological origins of the velar and laryngeal nerves (10th cranial nerve) explain why organic abnormalities in phonation and oral-nasal resonance balance are common. In addition, muscle misuses within the vocal tract often result in concurrent voice and resonance quality abberations: for example, hypertonicity in the tongue base may result not only in phonation limitations but also a degree of hypernasality because of a downward pull on the soft palate via hypertonic palatoglossus muscles.

A further possible origin of concurrent disorders of phonation and resonance relates to aerodynamic regulation/control mechanisms described by Warren [55, 56]. In instances of excessive or insufficient valving forces in the larynx or velopharyngeal port, one valve may compensate with greater or lesser closing forces in an attempt to regulate aerodynamic pressures so that they meet requirements for speech. For example, in cases of velopharyngeal valving incompetence and subsequent hypernasality in children with cleft palate, it is common to see hypervalving in the larynx. This laryngeal hypervalving may result in more appropriate intra-oral pressure levels for articulation, but may lead to dysphonia caused by the associated strain on the phonatory mechanism associated with long-term misuse.

Acoustic Analysis of Speech

From the voice-source spectrum, measures of frequency and amplitude perturbation (**jitter** and **shimmer** respectively), and signal-to-noise ratios in the acoustic spectrum may be used to supplement the voice quality assessment. Jitter and shimmer are measures of stability of the acoustic signal from one period to the next, and thus should reflect short-term stability of the phonatory mechanism (Figure 10.14, Chapter 10). Ratio measures of harmonic-to-noise energy indicate the degree to which the signal energy is periodic versus aperiodic and noisy. Both sustained vowel samples and recordings of connected speech may be analysed acoustically. A minimum protocol would include three trials of two different sustained vowels, one open and low, the other high and closed; and repetition or oral reading of a standard sentence which samples several different vowels and voiced segments, such as: 'I will be ready to go soon'. By making simultaneous digital acoustic recordings of phonation simultaneous with laryngostroboscopy, EGG and other measures of vibratory characteristics, the team can interpret more accurately the physical correlates of high jitter, shimmer or noise components from inverse-filtered signals of sustained vowels.

When acoustic measures are being used for pre- and post-treatment comparisons, it is critical that vocal production factors of intensity and frequency are controlled, since they influence perturbation and noise levels. Ideally, a natural discourse sample is also analysed, since articulatory contexts have been demonstrated to have an effect on glottic-source acoustic measures, and subsequent effects on vocal quality during speech should be identified [38]. Although a one-to-one correspondence does not exist between single acoustic measures and voice quality labels, in the case of certain perceptual measures, acoustic analysis of the signal may serve to validate and train listeners' judgements. For example, recent studies have demonstrated that voices judged to have high 'breathy/whispery' quality have acoustic spectra that include one or more of the following features: high levels of interharmonic noise, or replacement of harmonics by noise; regions of high-intensity noise in the spectra above the primary formants (6 kHz and higher); antiformants in the low-frequency spectra related to tracheal resonance; relatively high intensity in the fundamental harmonic (f_0) compared to that of adjacent harmonics, overall spectral energy, or the first formant [17, 29, 43, 47, 51] (Figure 10.13, Chapter 10). Sodersten, Lindestad and Hammarberg [51] have suggested that a differential acoustic profile may exist for breathiness associated with hypofunction compared with 'hyperfunctional' breathiness [51]. Careful examination of acoustic profiles may lead us to be more discriminating listeners, and to relate perceptual-acoustic features more precisely with phonatory behaviors.

The spectrum of the vocal tract transfer function may also be used to provide information about voice quality. By employing special algorithms (equations) some acoustical analysis programs allow the examiner to locate the frequency of the vocal tract resonances or formants for a given speech or phonation task. Formant features can provide information regarding changes in vocal tract postures, such as tongue, lip and jaw movements, or vocal tract lengthening and shortening. In the assessment of the singer's vocal technique, the location and intensity of formants can provide clues to the positioning of articulators, and may be used as a feedback tool in training.

Several caveats to interpretation of digital acoustic measures need to be considered. Firstly, recording equipment and environment, and A-to-D signal processing can influence the perturbation and noise values. In one study, different jitter and shimmer measures were derived for the same signals recorded with four different recording devices [15]. Clearly if one is to make valid and reliable comparisons, the recording equipment and environment must be calibrated carefully. Secondly, it is important to understand that many different algorithms (mathematical formulas) are represented in different software programs for acoustic analysis. Some are better suited to certain clinical measures than others, and it may not be meaningful to compare one with the other [41]. Further, acoustic measures may be based on either time or frequency domains. Even though time and frequency are inversely related in acoustic signals, they may not be equally meaningful for a given perturbation measure, such as jitter. Normative data employed as baseline measures against which to compare clinical data must be based on the same hardware, software, and tasks.

1.5 AERODYNAMIC EVALUATION

Clinical measures of phonatory flow rates and volumes, and intra-oral pressure and resistance allow the clinician to obtain information about glottic function in a non-invasive manner.

1.5.1 Mean Phonatory Flow Rate

Clinical measurement of flow rates during phonation is generally achieved with a full or partial face mask attached to a flow transducer unit (Figure 1.4). The device that transduces an aerodynamic to electric signal may be one of several types: pneumotachograph, hot-wire anemometer, plethysmograph, or electro-aerometer. The reader is referred to an excellent text on instrumental assessment by Baken for further details [4].

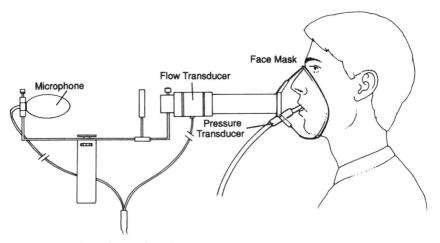

Figure 1.4 Hardware for aerodynamic assessment

Mean phonatory flow rates (MFR) measured on steady-state vowel productions provide estimates of glottic impedance, since resistance in the oral cavity is minimal compared to glottic resistance under this condition [4, 13]. Measures are usually quantified in milliliters per second or liters per second. Open vowel productions (for example, sustained /ɑ/) permit the most accurate estimate of laryngeal function to be obtained, since they generally offer the least resistance to phonatory flow. Normative data suggests a wide range of variability in this measure: from under 40 ml/s to over 300 ml/s in adults, and from approximately 50 ml/s to 170 ml/s in first-grade children [4, 10, 24]. The clinician is usually also interested in the effect that phonetic environment has on vocal function and, for this reason, aerodynamic measures should be made during connected speech samples under the most natural conditions possible (considering that the patient is often wearing a face mask). Sentences with a variety of contexts should be elicited, to determine the effect on MFR of voiceless versus voiced contexts, loud versus soft speech, different pitch ranges and other relevant vocal dynamics.

Phonatory flow rates have complex relationships with vocal intensity and fundamental frequency [25, 26]. For example, high intensity phonation at high f_0 levels is generally associated with high MFR, however the same relationship may not hold at lower f_0 levels. It is critical that production factors of f_0 and intensity be measured simultaneously with MFR, so that they can be controlled for reliability and averaging trials, and for pre- and post-treatment measures. This may be accomplished by time-locking separate acoustic measures with the aerodynamic recordings, or by using a dedicated device that records the acoustic and aerodynamic signals simultaneously. Because of the complex relationships with production factors, MFR measures should be made under a variety of intensity and frequency conditions during clinical assessment.

Other production factors held constant, high phonatory flow rates (for example, above 300 ml/s, in adult males, at normal speaking pitch and average loudness on /ɑ/) are indicative of poor glottic valving and subsequent DC leakage. This could be due to vocal fold weakness or paralysis; structural defects such as sulcus vocalis; lesions that inhibit complete vocal fold adduction; and other sources of glottic incompetence including those created by muscle misuse. Phonatory flow rates greater than 900 ml/s have been reported in individuals with recurrent laryngeal nerve paralysis [24], and in individuals phonating with an intentional posterior glottic chink [43]. Phonatory flow rates also tend to increase with longer open quotients in the vocal fold vibratory cycle. This vibratory feature may be a result of vocal technique, or reduced muscle tonus in the vocal folds. Low MFR rates (below 30 ml/s for adults, at speaking pitch and average loudness on /ɑ/) most often relate to muscle misuse behaviors that result in excessive vocal fold adductory forces and high medial compression. Low rates, however, have often been reported in well-trained singers [40]. Neurological conditions, such as laryngeal dystonia or Parkinson's disease may also contribute to hypervalving activity. If valving forces in the larynx are hyperkinetic then closed phase increases, amplitude of vibration decreases, and only small amounts of AC flow are released between the vocal folds during the open phase of the vibratory cycle. Lower intensity phonation is generally associated with lower phonatory flow rates. One example of a clinical exception to this rule would be higher flow rates associated with 'quieter' phonation in an individual who tends to hypervalve the glottis during 'louder' phonation, but relaxes the valve when lower intensity is required.

1.5.2 Flow Volume

Phonatory volume indicates the quantity of air that was exhaled during a given phonated segment, as measured with a pneumotachograph, flow transducer or other standard equipment, and quantified in liters or milliliters. As with phonatory flow rates, a wide range for normal function has been described. For adults on maximally sustained open vowels, ranges from 1520 to 2723 ml have been reported for females, and from

2200 to 4255 ml for males. The ranges for children reflect their smaller lung capacities: from 700 to 1650 ml (see [4, 24] for comprehensive reviews of normative data).

When phonatory flow measures are not available, they can be estimated by dividing phonatory volume by maximum phonation time. A less accurate, but nevertheless related estimate of flow rate can be obtained from the **phonation quotient** by dividing vital capacity measures by maximum phonation time [27, 59]. This value is generally somewhat higher than MFR values, since most individuals do not use their entire vital capacity during maximally sustained phonation [58].

1.5.3 Pressure and Resistance

Subglottic pressure and glottic resistance can be measured indirectly using the intra-oral method proposed by Smitheran and Hixon [49]. A small tube attached to a pressure transducer is placed between the lips so that its open end rests in the oral cavity, and can receive and transmit pressure changes to the transducer (Figure 1.4). This technique is based on the assumption that intra-oral pressure equals tracheal pressure when the glottis is open and the lips are sealed for production of a plosive consonant. The authors suggested repetition of /pi/ at a rate of 1.5 syllables per second, at habitual pitch and loudness for speech, with equal stress allotted to each syllable. Some clinicians feel a more representative speech pressure is obtained with an open vowel, so the syllable /pæ/ is elicited. Evidence suggests that pressure and resistance values are different for the syllables /pi/ and /pæ/, so the vowel should be controlled for intersubject and pre- and post-treatment comparisons [37]. Peak pressure values from /p/ productions can be measured and averaged across several successive productions (a minimum of 10 is recommended) to indicate mean subglottic pressure. Pressure values are traditionally made relative to water pressure, so clinical measures may be in centimeters of water (cm H_2O), or alternatively in dynes/cm^2.

Several precautions must be observed to ensure that valid measures are made with the intra-oral pressure technique. Firstly, the clinician's description and model of the syllable production must be presented in a manner that does not bias the patient's productions. A clear description of the task, and minimal modelling may elicit the most typical production from patients. An example of specific directions is: 'Now I would like you to say the sound /pipipi . . ./ repeatedly at your usual pitch and loudness level, at the speed I demonstrated. Say it as with your normal speech effort.' The goal is to elicit phonatory behavior that is indicative of an individual's typical speech behavior. As with phonatory flow measures, pressure varies with intensity and frequency values in speech. These must be carefully controlled when measures are being compared. Most normative data report average subglottic pressure values between 4.5 and 8 cm H_2O, as measured either from the indirect method described above, or directly from the subglottic space, by way of tracheal puncture. Lieberman [36] reported subglottic pressures in adults during speech that ranged from 5 to 10 cm H_2O.

Simultaneously-recorded phonatory flow measures (during the /i/ or /æ/ vowels) can be used in a simple equation to estimate average glottic resistance values:

Average glottic resistance = average glottic pressure (cm H_2O)/average flow rate (ml/s).

High glottic resistance values are expected in cases where glottic valving forces are exaggerated, and low values are associated with glottic valving incompetence.

1.5.4 Flow Glottograms

If clinical devices are available to obtain inverse-filtered phonatory flow measures, the resultant **flow glottogram** can provide useful details of vocal fold function [18]. Rothenberg [45, 46] designed a flow mask that performs the inverse filter function while phonation is recorded. The resulting signal is relatively free of vocal tract filter functions, so reflects primarily the aerodynamic characteristics related to vocal fold vibratory patterns. Values can be extracted from the signal for peak glottic flow, DC flow offset ('leakiness' factor), open, closed, and closing speed quotients. Simultaneous recordings of flow glottography and electroglottography demonstrate the inverse relationship between the signals as they represent the vocal fold vibratory pattern [23].

A sample protocol for aerodynamic assessment in the voice clinic is offered here. Several trials are recommended for each task so that values representing an individual's average performance can be calculated.

Protocol for aerodynamic assessment

1. Vital Capacity measure: maximum expiratory volume after maximum inhalation.
2. Sustained vowels /ɑ/; /i/, habitual pitch and loudness.
3. Sustained vowels /[ɑ/; /i/, high and low pitch and loudness compared with typical speech levels. *Hey* at various loudness levels.
4. Maximum phonation time on vowels (for phonation quotient calculations, as necessary).
5. f_0 Dynamics: slow glissando up/down throughout entire range. Vary intensity with different trials.
6. Speech samples: 'Tell me your name, occupation, and one other thing about yourself'; 'Count from one to ten'; 'Count from eleven to twenty'. (These could be used to examine consonant devoicing effects on vowel MFR).

Say these sentences (model verbally, or have patient read from a cue card): 'Please, seat Shelly, Harriet and Frederick close to the fire' (look at coarticulatory devoicing effect on MFR of vowels); 'Are you really angrier than you were on Monday?' (look at MFR in absence of devoicing effect).

7. 'Say /pæ pæ pæ pæ . . ./ at this speed (1.5 syllables per second), using your usual pitch and loudness. Say it with your normal speaking effort.' (for pressure (/p/) and flow (/æ/) measures, and calculation of laryngeal resistance: resistance = pressure/flow).
8. Therapy probes.

1.6 MUSCULOSKELETAL EVALUATION

All members of the voice care team are involved in assessing postural and muscle misuse tendencies in our patients. Since voluntary muscles are the final common pathway for psychological and physiological function during speech and singing, it is of primary importance to identify specific muscle misuse patterns contributing to dysphonias. The musculoskeletal evaluation begins during the history interview, when both the interviewer and observers take note of static postural profiles, and changes in posture that may occur with changes in topic. General observations such as 'slouching' or 'overstraightened' may be used to describe initial clinical impressions. Since the history interview is the clinical protocol that may elicit the most natural discourse from patients, it is important to document more specific postural misuses as precisely as possible. These observations may be augmented during discussions with the psychiatrist, speech pathologist and singing teacher, with each team member noting specific situations, topics or voice features that correspond with particular muscle misuse patterns.

It would be an oversight to suggest that postural abnormalities are always related to muscle misuse and/or psychogenic factors: a variety of structural disorders and neurological disease processes may result in abnormal muscle tone, or misalignment and asymmetry that may contribute to speech and voice dysfunction. Patients with such disorders may show limited responses to the traditional therapy programs for posture retraining. Nevertheless, behavioral or habitual muscle misuse remains the most common cause of postural abnormalities.

Postural misuses that may be observed and quantified during the initial interview and subsequent assessment activities are discussed below.

1.6.1 Indicators of Body Misalignment

As part of the postural pattern, the scapulae may be adducted, so that the shoulders are positioned unnaturally posteriorly, and power in the upper arms is disengaged (Figure 1.5a).

If the back and neck muscles are being misused, a 'hump' may be observable in the upper back, just below the cervical vertebrae. Misuse of the neck muscles can lead to hyperextension or flexion of the neck (Figure 1.5b). Commonly, the head is retracted on the neck, so that the jaw extends up and forward, a misuse we refer to as **jaw jut**. The opposite postural misuse is also observed, although not as often: where the head is held forward with neck flexion. It is important to inquire about injuries that may have contributed to postural misuse, in particular, a history of whiplash injuries. The head–neck posture may reflect attempts by some individuals to compensate for poorly fitting spectacles, or other visual acuity problems.

During respiration, the abdomen may be held tightly in conjunction with hypertonicity in the pelvic floor muscles. In this situation, exaggerated inspiratory movements in the rib cage and auxiliary movements of the clavicles may be observed. These areas may also be inappropriately held in the inspiratory position to exaggerated

Figure 1.5 Body misalignment and muscle misuses.

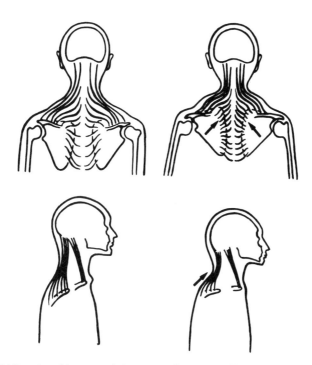

Figure 1.5 (a) Scapulae adduction and elevation (right, upper and lower) compared with normal use (left, upper and lower).

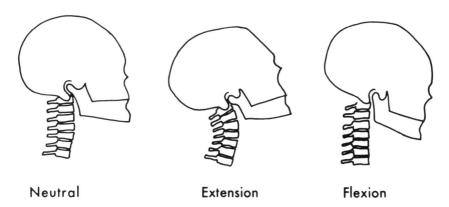

Neutral   Extension   Flexion

Figure 1.5 (b) inappropriate neck postures: hyper-extension ('jaw jut') (center); hyperflexion (right), compared with normal use (left).

degrees during exhalation and phonation. In the absence of free respiratory movements, additional auxiliary inspiratory tactics may be observed including head retraction (jaw jut) and tongue retraction. A 'hands-on' approach to assessment of respiratory function provides useful supplementary information: with the examiners hands on the abdomen and back; and then on lateral portions of the rib cage, he/she feels for evidence of the appropriate abdomen/lower rib cage distension during inspiration at rest, and preparatory to various phonatory tasks. By palpating the submental region just anterior to the hyoid bone, the examiner can detect inappropriate muscle activity in the suprahyoid muscles during inspiration, which are associated with tongue retraction, and sometimes jaw extension.

1.6.2 Specific Muscle Misuses During Phonation

A common misuse of respiratory muscles during phonation, especially for vocal performance, is failure to support the lung volume with inspiratory muscle activity once phonation has been initiated (Figure 1.5c). This is a function of poor body posture and technical misuse. At high lung volumes especially, the intrinsic inspiratory muscles, in particular the external intercostals, need to be engaged during phonation so that subglottic pressure does not exceed requirements for the voice task. In instances where subglottic pressure is allowed to exceed the optimal level, the laryngeal muscles may respond by valving to decelerate the airflow at the glottis, which results in excessive glottic compression. Further adjustments in the larynx may be made to allow for continued phonation, for example, contraction of the inspiratory posterior crico-arytenoid muscles may create a posterior glottic chink which acts as a pressure-release valve, while medial compression is maintained in the anterior portions of the vocal folds for phonation.

Misuse of muscles governing movements at the temporomandibular joint (TMJ) are common. The lower facial muscles may be hypertonic, so minimal or no jaw movement is noted during speech. If the lateral pterygoid and buccinator muscles are contracted, the mandible may be held forward or pulled forward during opening gestures (Figure 1.5d). With the head of the mandible disengaged from the glenoid fossa and articular capsule, free rotational movements are no longer possible. Thus mandible depression is reduced and any movements observed during speech are stiff. To assess tension in mandible elevators in a nonvocal situation, the examiner attempts to rotate the jaw with his/her hand. With the examiner's hands placed flat over the TMJ region, 'bulging' during speech or jaw depression can be felt if exaggerated or inappropriate forward movements are being made.

Further misuse of the tongue/jaw complex may be evidenced by palpation of the suprahyoid muscles during inspiratory and phonatory tasks (Figure 1.5e). Of particular significance is persistent hypertonicity in the suprahyoids during speech and singing; increased activity during inspiration; increased activity in association with pitch or loudness dynamics. Often, in untrained or poorly trained singers, the suprahyoid muscles are noted to become increasingly hypertonic with rising pitch, and around register transitions. The larynx may be pulled upward with this muscle misuse, as

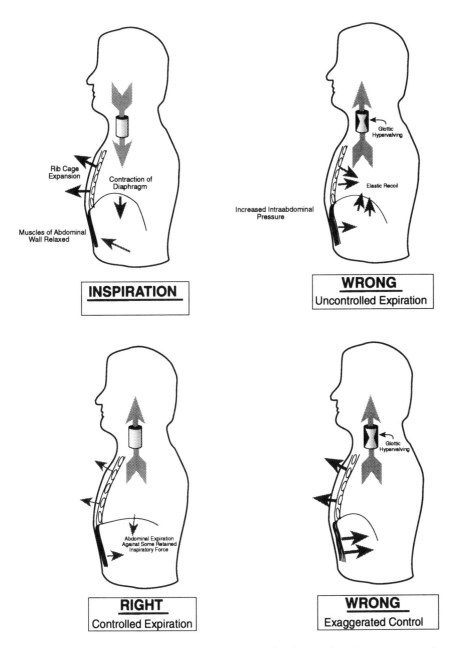

Figure 1.5 (c) misuses of the respiratory system compared with normal use for inspiration and expiration.

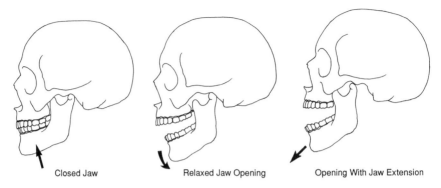

Closed Jaw   Relaxed Jaw Opening   Opening With Jaw Extension

Figure 1.5 (d) misuse of the temporomandibular joint: forward extension during opening, compared with normal use for speech.

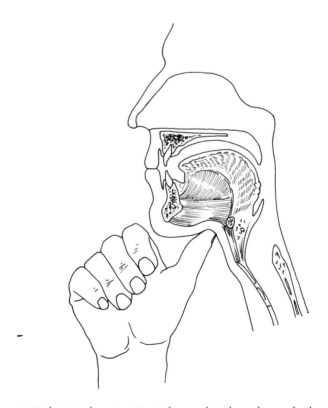

Figure 1.5 (e) detecting hypertonicity in the suprahyoid muscle complex by palpation.

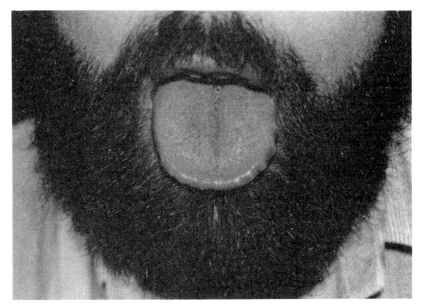

Figure 1.5 (f) tongue scalloping due to hypertonicity in tongue muscles 'at rest': tongue pushes forward into the lower teeth, leaving an imprint of the teeth on the tongue periphery.

confirmed by laryngoscopy, or by palpation of the thyroid cartilage during scales and glissando pitch changes. Abnormal tongue posturing and muscle tone may be associated with mild hypernasality, due to involvement of the palatoglossus muscle: when hypertonic, this muscle may cause lowering of the soft palate, thus reducing the adequacy of the velopharyngeal closure during speech. Further, if the tongue is held posterior to its rest position so it reduces the pharyngeal space, oropharyngeal resonance may be damped, and excessive nasal resonance may be noted due to increased flow through the nasal cavity. Not surprisingly, many individuals with muscle misuse voice disorders also exhibit abnormal resonance features.

If the tongue muscles are hypertonic at rest, the periphery of the tongue may have a 'scalloped' appearance, an imprint made by the lower teeth as the tongue is pressed against them for long periods. (Figure 1.5f) Conversely, the tongue may be held in a retracted position at rest, so the edges do not rest against the bottom teeth. Observation of the surface of the tongue at rest and on protrusion may reveal excessive narrowing and grooving indicative of intrinsic muscle tension, and the tongue surface may tremor inconsistently at rest.

Laryngeal posture at rest and during phonation is of importance to phonatory function, and can be assessed informally by palpating the thyroid notch. The vertical position of the larynx following a swallow may be used as a reference point for rest. Exaggerated excursion of the larynx during speech or singing (more than a few millimetres) is suspect, as is a phonatory posture superior to the rest position. Some singing styles appear to be enhanced by a laryngeal position that is slightly lower than the post-swallow rest position. In this case, it is important that the singing posture for the larynx is not maintained after the phonatory activity is completed, so the muscles lowering the larynx are not chronically hypertonic. Detailed evaluation of a variety of laryngeal postures is made using the flexible transnasal fiberoptic scope which permits observation of the larynx during speech and nonspeech activities. This technique is discussed in the next section.

The functions of the facial muscles are many and varied. Beyond its perceptual, respiratory and deglutition functions, the face serves as a platform for revealing prevailing conscious or unconscious emotions, and the intent behind communicative gestures such as speech. This may explain why facial muscles are so susceptible to misuse. The freedom of speech and voice movements can be jeopardized by tension in muscles in the upper, mid, and lower face areas. Observe signs of anxiety, depression, and/or denial in the upper face: eyebrows elevated or adducted; cheeks elevated; gaze fixed for long periods. In the lower face, the lips may be pressed together at rest, the upper lip retracted and virtually immobile during speech, the jaw immobile during speech, the mentalis muscles of the chin puckered, all signs of muscle misuse which may be indicative of ongoing emotional distress. If upper and lower facial postures are functioning to inhibit emotional expression, then the specific muscle misuses governing movements of the lips, jaw and tongue during phonation may be fairly easy to identify, but difficult to treat without psychiatric intervention.

1.7 PHYSICAL EXAMINATION OF THE LARYNX AND VOCAL TRACT

1.7.1 Basic Equipment Needs

The otolaryngologist's examination with a head mirror and laryngeal mirror remains the clinical standard, and coupled with a full head and neck examination is the way that the vast majority of voice disordered patients are assessed. But clinically useful information is obtainable with rigid and flexible fiberoptic instruments particularly when they are attached to a video camera, and this section focuses on the type of set-up that we use in our clinic.

Hardware equipment systems for a voice clinic set-up evolve rapidly and, as with computers, one always wants to have next year's model. The key elements include:

Light source

Reliable halogen lights are available without spending too much money. Expensive xenon arc lamps are not necessary since the quality of light sensitive video cameras has increased.

Flexible fiberoptic laryngoscope

Several excellent models are available and the important variables include the diameter of the instrument, the amount of light transmitted, and the magnification offered when connected to the camera. Pediatric models are usually slimmer and easier to pass but may sacrifice brightness and image size.

Rigid glass rod laryngoscope

As with the above, the brightness, ease of focusing, size and clarity of image are paramount. The main difference between available models is in the light beam angulation at the tip, with both 70° and 90° scopes being offered. To some extent the difference comes down to personal preference and experience. Some of the 90° laryngoscopes have a focusing ring that permits a wider aperture lens and therefore more available light, but it is sometimes fussy to get a sharply focused image. It is probably a good idea to get an instrument that has the fiberoptic cable permanently attached to the telescope, as the detachable junction provides a zone for damage and light loss.

Video camera

The evolution of technology during the past decade in this part of the field has been truly amazing, and it will undoubtedly continue. It is still possible to attach the scopes to a C-mount on an inexpensive home video camera, but the size, clarity, and cost features of cameras designed to attach to an endoscope have improved to the point that low-cost compromises may be false economy. Yanigasawa has kept us abreast of how these changes relate to assessment of voice disorders, and those in the market for a system would do well to find his latest update [57].

Stroboscope

Strobed light has been used to examine the larynx for a great many years, but it was not until the image could be recorded on video that its tremendous value in the clinic was realized. There are four or five instrument companies that market excellent strobe generators specially designed for laryngeal examination. The fundamental frequency of vocal fold vibration is detected by a neck stethoscope, and the light generated by the machine is turned on and off and modulated in various ways by a foot control.

Audio microphone

A relatively inexpensive lapel-mounted electret microphone is used for most situations but it may be desirable to use a unidirectional headset-mounted microphone to maintain high fidelity and a constant distance if the recordings are also used for a computerized acoustic analysis or perceptual-acoustic ratings.

Video recorder

In 1980 we began to make all of our recordings on $\frac{3}{4}$ inch (19 mm) tape, using 20-minute cassettes. This provided us with a satisfactory combination of quality, ease of retrieval, editability, and portability since most meeting sites and educational venues used that format. This has changed. Excellent Super VHS machines have the advantage of high quality with a smaller format, and since the rewind speed is so much greater we can get many more patient recordings on one tape. Additionally, these units have built in editing facilities and three or more input ports so that more than one camera or video recorder can be interconnected without the need for extra switch assemblies.

It is useful to have an inexpensive home video camera mounted in the clinic room in such a way as to allow for a quick switch from the endoscopic recordings to a video-recorded interview to document the various aspects of voice function.

Video monitor

Models are available that can show an increased number of lines of resolution and thereby make good use of the extra benefits of Super VHS recording.

Storage of equipment

A cart with drawers for all the bits of paraphernalia is a great help. Tissues, gauze, defoggers, cleaning solutions, biopsy forceps, gloves, anaesthetic spray, tongue depressors, etc. all need a place.

It is best if all of these components can be dedicated to the voice clinic area, so that as the patient is being assessed they are all there ready to be turned on. It is also practical if they can be mounted on a sturdy but movable cart. Storage of equipment on wall shelving can be cumbersome because most of the cables connect on the back of each machine.

1.7.2 Regional Examination

Tongue and oral cavity

The tongue and its movements and the oral cavity mucosa are examined for presence of lesions or evidence of neurological disorders. During an oral mechanism exam, indicators of certain muscle misuse patterns can also be identified, such as tongue scalloping or jaw and tongue tension.

Larynx and pharynx

In the past, physical examination of the larynx was the primary responsibility of the laryngologist, who would report the observations and interpretations to other professionals involved in caring for a patient. The ability to document the laryngoscopic examination on videotape, show the patient his or her own larynx, and interpret the findings with other professionals such as the speech pathologist or singing teacher is the principal reason that voice clinic teams have evolved, and that there has been so much interest in voice and advances in our understanding of voice disorders.

Mirror examination of the larynx is the standard in most otolaryngology offices, and shall remain so with good reason. We will not spend time discussing this technique here since it does not offer the multi-observer advantage of video endoscopes. Video imaging of the larynx during endoscopy using the flexible fiberoptic transnasal technique, or transoral endoscopy with a rigid telescope does allow multiple observers to view and evaluate laryngeal function.

What are the advantages of flexible fiberoptic endoscopy over use of the rigid telescope? Briefly, the flexible scope is best for 'macrolaryngoscopy' and the rigid for 'microlaryngoscopy'. A transnasal observation of the entire upper vocal tract is essential for a full evaluation of connected speech and laryngeal postures, particularly during evaluation of muscle misuse voice disorders (Figure 1.6a). Some of the supraglottic postures described in the chapter on classification (Chapter 2) went unrecognized until laryngeal examination could be readily achieved without pulling on the tongue. Since examination with the flexible scope does not need to interfere with articulatory movements in the oral cavity, (although it may affect velopharyngeal closure on the side of insertion) it provides a distinct advantage for the documentation of connected speech samples. Examination with the rigid endoscope generally involves tongue protrusion, and is restricted to phonation on a vowel that is associated with

Figure 1.6 Techniques for indirect laryngoscopic examination.

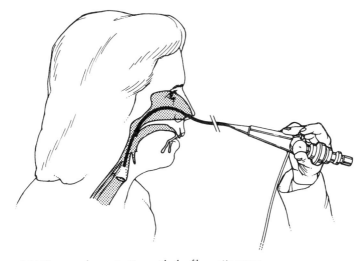

Figure 1.6 (a) Transnasal examination with the fibreoptic scope.

anterior tongue placement (usually /i/; *ee*) that makes the larynx more visually accessible.

A bonus afforded by the emergence of flexible transnasal fiberoscopy is an excellent view of the nose and nasopharynx. By using this technique routinely with voice disordered patients we have found unexpected pathology, particularly in the nasopharynx, that may have been related to the problem in question but have gone undetected in a standard mirror exam. Inflamed cysts or bursae are examples. There are still those 'gaggers' that cannot be seen by any method other than from direct examination under general anesthetic, which one would obviously like to avoid and which provides no useful information regarding speech behavior.

A tendency for those performing indirect laryngoscopy on a patient is to seek a view through the pharynx and supraglottic structures to the vocal folds, and then ignore all else. Chapter 2 highlights the clinical significance of static and dynamic aspects of glottic and supraglottic postures including false-cord adduction and anteroposterior contraction of supraglottic structures. If you are fortunate to be able to videorecord the examination then you may keep the document and discuss it further after other factors, such as psychological ones, have been considered. In any event you must make a conscious effort to evaluate the supraglottic structures before passing on to a close view of vocal fold activity.

While the flexible exam gives the best overview, the rigid telescope with its clarity of optics and great magnification is the best for looking at the details of vocal fold structure. (Figure 1.6b) The features we seek to examine with the strobe light such as glottic closure, phase, mucosal wave, viscosity, discrimination between cysts [8] and nodules, etc. are all displayed to the best advantage with rigid videolaryngoscopy. The effects of altering head and neck posture during the laryngeal examination must be considered in the final interpretation of clinical data obtained. Sodersten and Lindestad [50] noted significant differences in laryngeal closure patterns associated with laryngostroboscopy using the flexible versus rigid laryngoscope, in particular, the perceived magnitude of posterior glottic chinks was larger in recordings made with the transoral rigid technique. This finding may be related to the typical posture adopted by patients to facilitate an easy view of the larynx. If the laryngoscope is placed centrally in the mouth, the patient's head must generally be retracted, and this may serve to bias laryngeal posture and affect vibratory patterns.

We have found that lateral placement of the laryngoscope allows for an excellent view of the vocal folds to be obtained without neck extension (Figure 1.6c). The scope can be pivoted on the first or second molar for stability, and the angle of the image corrected by rotating the camera at its attachment to the laryngoscope. Figure 1.6 demonstrates the effects of two different positions of the rigid scope on the laryngeal view, and the head–neck postures associated with each examination approach.

Since different types of information can be gleaned from flexible and rigid laryngoscopy, both techniques are essential for a comprehensive clinical examination. Both continuous and flashing (stroboscopic) light sources may be used to obtain visual perceptual information regarding anatomical and physiological status of the larynx during phonation.

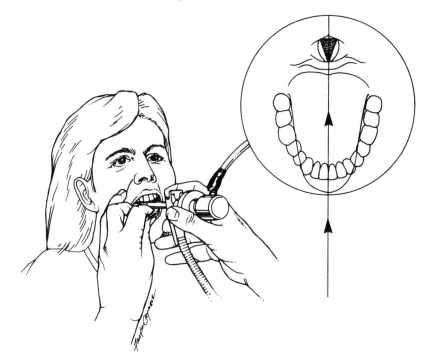

Figure 1.6 (b) Transoral examination with the rigid laryngoscope; frontal placement.

1.7.3 Instrumental Assessment of Vocal Fold Vibratory Patterns

During indirect and direct examination of the larynx, a continuous light source is generally used to examine gross structural and movement characteristics. This examination technique is supplemented in the modern-day voice clinic by use of a flashing 'stroboscopic' light source coupled with fiberoptic or telescopic hardware and video-audio recording devices.

Phonatory parameters measured with continuous light

Rate, range and symmetry of abduction and adduction movements
The rate and excursion of lateral vocal fold movements for nonspeech tasks such as normal and deep inspiration, and vegetative adduction during coughing, swallowing, or gagging provides information about the functional status of the crico-arytenoid joint and the muscles that govern movement from that joint. Slow, incoordinate, asymmetrical or reduced movements may indicate central or peripheral neurological disease, fixation, or dislocation of the crico-arytenoid joint.

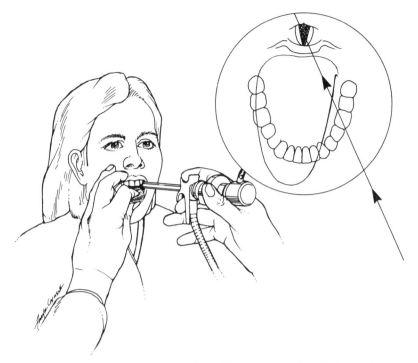

Figure 1.6 (c) transoral examination with the rigid laryngoscope; lateral placement.

Laryngeal diadochokinesis
This evaluates the rate of repetition of the vowel /i/, and the syllable /hi/ that requires the 'devoicing' gesture for voiceless articulations in speech. The normal ranges in adults are 4–7 repetitions per second [6]. Rates below norm may indicate central or neurological disease, fixation of the crico-arytenoid joint or laryngeal muscle hypertonicity.

Glottic and supraglottic postures
This includes the general relationships of laryngeal structures to each other during phonation and at rest. During phonation, we assess the degree of anterior–posterior and lateral compression of the supraglottic structures, and the phonatory closure patterns at the glottis elicited with a wide variety of speech tasks. Posture patterns outlined in Chapter 2 provide a guideline for assessment of glottic and supraglottic postures. Closure patterns are assessed in greater detail for sustained vowels with the stroboscopic light.

Vocal fold edges
This implies the straightness and smoothness of the medial edges of each vocal fold. Lesions, scarring, and other organic problems can result in irregular margins.

Stroboscopic evaluation

Video-stroboscopic techniques have been used in routine voice evaluation for over a decade. The principles of stroboscopic imaging are based on perceptual features of the optical system. The human visual system is temporally limited in its ability to perceive more than about five images per second. Since the vocal folds vibrate at much higher speeds than this during phonation (100–1000 vibrations per second) the examiner is not equipped to distinguish details of movement patterns associated with each vibratory cycle. The stroboscope provides a flashing light source that can solve this perceptual dilemma in the examination of phonatory patterns.

The fundamental frequency of vocal fold vibration (f_0) is detected by a microphone placed on the anterior neck, and this information is transmitted to the stroboscope to drive the light generator. By flashing at approximately the same frequency as the f_0 of vocal fold vibration, the stroboscopic light illuminates a single image of each vibratory cycle. The visual system then takes over by creating an 'averaged' image of the vocal fold vibratory pattern over many cycles (Figure 1.7a and b). If the stroboscopic light is set to flash at exactly the same frequency as the vocal f_0, the optical image is of a constant phase of the vibratory cycle, for example the beginning of closing (Figure 1.7b). This setting allows the examiner to perceive the averaged degree of irregularity or aperiodicity from one cycle to the next.

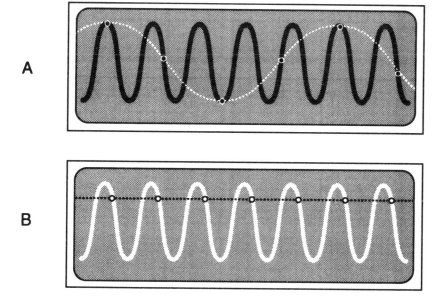

Figure 1.7 Principles of stroboscopy: (a) if the light is set to flash slightly off the f_0, a slow-motion image will be perceived; (b) if the light is set to flash at the same frequency as f_0 ('phase-locked'), the image will give the impression of a still-frame.

A different setting will allow the stroboscopic light to be driven at a frequency several hertz different from the f_0, thus illuminating the vocal folds at a slightly different phase than f_0, as seen in Figure 1.7a. This allows for a 'slow-motion' visual effect that gives the perceiver an impression of the approximate or average movement pattern of successive vibratory cycles. Although the visual perception created by this system is not as accurate as slow-motion photographic images, it is a much easier and faster clinical procedure. Unless the vibratory cycles are extremely irregular, stroboscopic imaging seems to provide a good approximation to the pattern of single, successive vibratory cycles for a given phonatory task [7, 28].

Because of their superior quality, we favour telescopic images viewed from the transoral rigid endoscope for our detailed stroboscopic evaluation. This hardware limits the speech task to approximation of a target /i/ vowel, and may involve holding the tongue forward to give adequate visual access to the larynx. Wherever possible, the lateral scope placement is used to minimize the need for neck extension and, if the larynx can be visualized well without holding the tongue, the patient is requested to position his tongue forward during the exam. Despite the obvious speech limitations, we feel that by recording a wide variety of vocal tasks, the examiner can gain a good understanding of the range of phonatory function related to vocal fold vibratory patterns. A sample clinical protocol for videostroboscopic examination is provided below.

Phonatory parameters measured with stroboscopic light

The following parameters related to vocal fold vibratory characteristics are measured perceptually from the videostroboscopic recordings.

Amplitude
The extent of vertical–lateral excursion of the vocal folds (Figure 1.8a) is the amplitude. With stroboscopy, amplitude is rated as lateral displacement from the glottic midline. Greatest amplitude is seen during loud phonation in modal register unless this is accompanied by laryngeal constriction. Reduced vibratory amplitude during phonation at typical speaking pitch and effort levels is related to excessive or reduced glottic valving, low subglottic pressure, vocal fold stiffness, and/or poor respiratory support.

Amplitude symmetry
This is the degree to which amplitude is the same for each vocal fold regardless of phase symmetry. Amplitude asymmetry may indicate greater stiffness (due to scarring or tension, or both), flaccidity (due to denervation), or mass (due to lesions) on one vocal fold.

Glottic closure pattern
The overall shape of closure during the most closed phase of phonation is known as the glottic closure pattern (Figure 1.8b). Possible descriptors for this characteristic include:

- complete;

Figure 1.8 Some phonatory parameters measured with stroboscopic light.

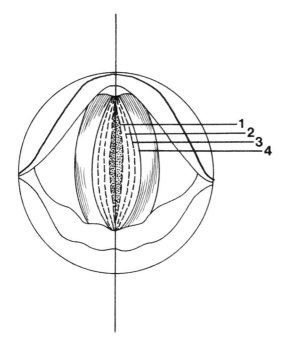

Figure 1.8 (a) Amplitude of vibrations: from small (most medial position) to large (most lateral position). Symmetry of amplitude should also be noted.

- posterior chink (commonly associated with muscle misuse, but also seen on a smaller scale in female adults without voice complaints);
- anterior chink (usually related to a structural defect);
- anterior and posterior chink ('hourglass' – commonly associated with bilateral nodules);
- irregular chink (often associated with irregular vocal fold edges, scarring and/or lesions);
- bowed folds ('spindle-shaped'—associated with neurogenic, psychogenic, muscle misuse or aging processes);
- incomplete closure along the entire length of the vocal fold margins (commonly associated with paralysis or psychogenic conversion aphonias).

The glottic closure may be rated further by degree using an equal-appearing interval scale, or descriptors: 'mild'; 'moderate'; 'severe'.

Mucosal wave
The mucosal wave is the extent of the travelling wave on the vocal fold mucosal cover (Figure 1.8c). This can be seen as a line or horizontal light travelling from the medial to

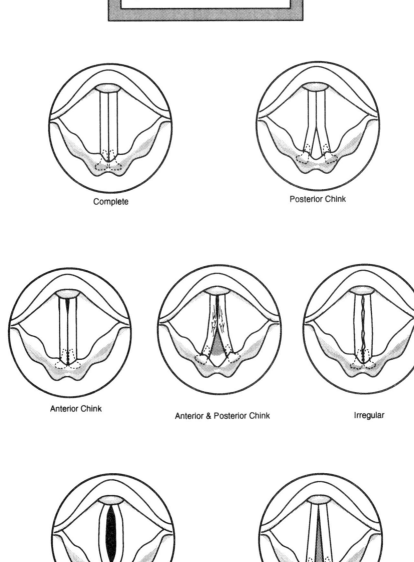

Figure 1.8 (b) glottic closure patterns during phonation.

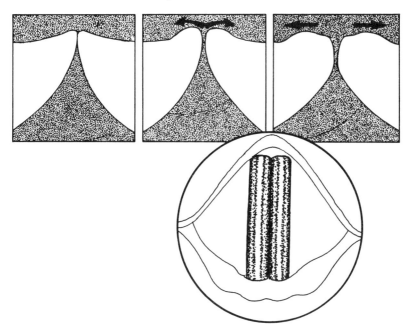

Figure 1.8 (c) mucosal wave: the perception of a 'travelling wave' from medial to lateral on the surface of the vocal folds.

the lateral surface of the vocal folds. It is most evident during loud phonation in modal register unless this is accompanied by laryngeal constriction. It is not always easy to decide whether or not an immobile vocal fold is paralysed or not. Stroboscopic examination can be helpful in determining the presence of motor tone, or reveal the gradual return of tone during recovery, by observation of the mucosal wave during phonation. The wave is dependant on a different tissue viscosity between the mucosal cover and muscle. The atonic flaccid cord tends to flap in the breeze like a flag. Think of it as 'flaccid flap'. Tissue scarring that results in tethering of the mucosa to deep lamina propria or muscle layers, and mass-altering lesions, may also result in reduced mucosal wave.

Phase closure
The ratio of open-to-closed phase during the averaged vibratory cycle is the phase closure. This can be estimated from the recorded video image by counting the number of video frames for the most closed phase of several successive cycles, the number of frames for the complete cycle, and calculating a separate mean ratio for each condition of phonation examined. Phase closure may vary considerably with pitch and loudness conditions so should be estimated separately for each task. Closed phase duration may be reduced by conditions limiting medial compression or arytenoid adduction, such as decreased muscle tone, large posterior glottic chinks, or paralysis. Closed phase

duration may be increased by hyperkinetic behavior such as excessive laryngeal valving due to muscle misuse and psychopathology.

Phase symmetry

Phase symmetry is the degree to which the vocal fold excursions represent mirror images of each other regardless of amplitude symmetry (Figure 1.8d). To perceive asymmetrical function one asks: Is one vocal fold leading in the opening/closing phases? Is one opening while the other is closing? (180° out of phase). Although amplitude symmetry and phase symmetry are evaluated separately, in reality they often coexist, and this makes the independent perceptual judgements more difficult. Unequal vocal fold mass, muscle tone or posture may result in phase asymmetry.

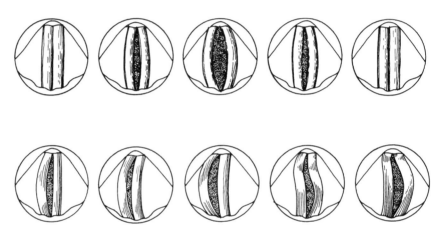

Figure 1.8 (d) phase symmetry (upper)/asymmetry (lower): degree to which the vocal fold movements represent mirror images of each other with respect to rate of opening and closing.

Regularity/periodicity

This is the degree to which successive averaged oscillatory cycles resemble each other. This is assessed in phase-locked setting, that is when the strobe is driven at the same frequency as the vocal fundamental frequency so that the same part of the phase is sampled for each perceptual image. In the video image the degree to which the image remains still or 'jitters' reflects the degree of regularity/irregularity (Figure 1.8e). It is important to assess the degree of variability in this characteristic based on pitch, loudness and posture. Irregularity or aperiodicity in the vocal fold vibratory patterns should relate closely to measures of perturbation in the glottic source acoustic waveform. Phase asymmetry may confound the perceptual judgments of regularity/ irregularity especially if phase-locked setting is not used.

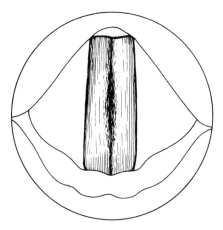

Figure 1.8 (e) irregularity/aperiodicity: degree to which the averaged cycles resemble each other, as measured with phase-locked light flashes: in this case the visual image is 'blurred' because successive cycles are different.

Vertical level of vocal fold approximation
This is the degree to which the vocal folds appear to adduct in the same or different horizontal plane for phonation. If a discrepancy exists between the vocal fold levels during adduction, closure and vibratory characteristics may be affected to varying degrees. Vocal fold approximation that is 'off-plane' may be related to unilateral paralysis, dystonia, dislocation of the crico-arytenoid joint or laryngeal injury.

Viscosity/stiffness
This is a clinical judgement of the degree to which the vocal folds are not vibrating under normal phonatory conditions. This parameter depends on a cumulative perceptual impression based on amplitude, mucosal wave, and symmetry ratings. Stiffness may be symmetrical or asymmetrical, and may be related to muscle hypertonicity, scarring, or other lesions. With the possible exception of hypertonicity, these conditions will have a pervasive influence on stiffness judgments under all pitch, loudness and posture conditions.

Protocol for video laryngostroboscopic assessment
The following is a list of tasks to be performed and recorded during laryngoscopic examination for comprehensive evaluation of vocal fold vibratory patterns. Several trials are recommended for each task so that values representing an individual's average performance can be calculated.

With continuous light source
- regular, quiet respiration

- deep inspiration
- cough, swallow
- connected speech, singing
- loud/soft speech, singing
- sustained phonation on vowels
- glissando pitch changes.

With stroboscopic light source (target phoneme is /i/):

- Sustained phonation: within habitual speaking pitch and loudness range. Include stroboscopic settings for apparent motion (frequency different from f_0) and phase-locked (frequency $= f_0$).
- Pitch glissandos on sustained phonation: slowly ascending and descending pitch to demonstrate maximum range parameters and all register transitions.
- High and low pitched sustained phonation: target several different pitches above and below habitual speaking pitch range.
- High and low intensity phonation: request 'loud' and 'soft' voice compared with habitual speaking loudness range.
- Sustained inhalation phonation: especially useful to identify muscle misuse components of habitual phonation which may not be present during inhalation phonation.
- Probe therapy: to determine potential for change with therapy techniques, for example: cough, push, nasalize sound, phonation with reduced lung volume, inhalation phonation to effect more complete closure; or sigh, relax to reduce hyperadduction behaviors. (Section 1.9 gives further details.)

Biasing effects

Although a comprehensive assessment requires that all relevant data on history, physical status and other instrumental measures be obtained, the examiners must appreciate the biasing power that pre-determined information may have on their perceptual evaluations. It is conceivable that objective measures of voice function and aspects of medical and psychological history will influence the acoustic and/or visual perceptual judgments of pre-informed examiners [42, 53]. A recent study demonstrated that the strongest examiner biasing effects during stroboscopy ratings were evident for least experienced examiners, and for subjects who had mild or moderate aberrations of vocal fold structure and function [53]. In light of the evidence for examiner bias, it is advisable to have acoustic and stroboscopy recordings rated by experienced clinicians who are not informed of a patient's history and phonatory function data, so the most reliable perceptual judgments can be obtained.

Electroglottography

EGG is a device for measuring changes in electrical impedance of the glottis, or the degree to which a high-frequency (but low-voltage) electric current passes between the two vocal folds. This is accomplished by means of two or more electrodes placed on the surface of the neck external to the larynx, with one over each thyroid lamina. Since human tissue conducts the current very well, but air does not, the degree of impedance is constantly changing with the degree of contact between the two vocal folds during phonation. Thus, aspects of the vocal fold contact area can be illustrated on a cycle-to-cycle basis. Perhaps the greatest clinical value derived from EGG recordings thus far is the extraction of f_0. Unless a vocal signal is very aperiodic, the rate of repetition of signals recorded with EGG provides an accurate and reliable representation of vocal f_0 [5]. On the other hand, the amplitude of the signal during the high-impedance ('open') phase is not directly related to acoustic amplitude or intensity. A multichannel EGG system has been introduced that reduces measurement artifacts and thus more accurately represents vocal fold contact area [44].

Recently, investigators have begun to combine EGG with other measures of vocal fold vibratory patterns [3, 9, 16, 23, 35]. As a result, guidelines for interpretation of the EGG signal are evolving, and its usefulness and limitations are becoming better understood [54]. As EGG equipment methodology and interpretation are improved we are able to derive more clinically relevant information from the signals. However certain precautions and caveats still need to be observed for this measure to be used in clinical decision making [11]. Figure 1.9 demonstrates the placement of EGG electrodes and the nature of the resultant waveform.

Photoglottography

Whereas electroglottography provides information about vocal fold contact area, and is thus based on the closing/closed phases of phonation, photoglottography (PGG) takes advantage of the degree of opening during phonation by measuring the amount of light that is transmitted through the vocal folds at any given time. PGG is a more invasive procedure than EGG, since a light and light sensor must be placed in opposition to each other, one above and one below the larynx (Figure 1.9). This probably explains why PGG is used less frequently in voice evaluation.

Typically the light source for a transoral or transnasal endoscope may be used, although a recent study reported success with placement of a high-intensity flashlight in the mouth [19]. A surface light sensor may be placed in the region of the cricothyroid membrane to detect the light during glottic opening, or a sensor may be suspended under the glottis through the interarytenoid space. Photoglottography provides the raw material to make temporal estimates of vocal fold vibratory patterns, including time of opening/closing, opening/open quotients and speed quotients. As with EGG, it provides the most useful details of phonatory function when combined with other simultaneously recorded clinical measures, such as stroboscopy, EGG, and inverse filtering of acoustic or flow signals.

Flow glottography

The inverse-filtered flow signal provides specific information about vocal fold vibratory

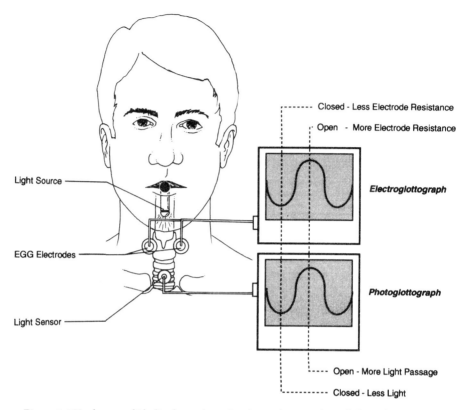

Figure 1.9 Hardware and idealized waveforms for electroglottography and photoglottography.

patterns, and is therefore an instrumental measure relevant to this section. Its use is discussed briefly in section 1.5

Laryngeal electromyography

It is our impression that, at this time, laryngeal electromyography (EMG) serves three functions. Firstly it can be used as a diagnostic tool to determine the state of innervation of selected muscles and has value in the management of some cases of laryngeal paralysis. For example, the presence or absence of normal cricothyroid muscle activity may help to differentiate between vagal and recurrent laryngeal nerve paralysis; and re-innervation signals may be prognostically useful when making management decisions in some cases of recurrent paralysis. Secondly, EMG recordings provide a very useful guide to needle placement during transcutaneous injection of botulinum toxin for spasmodic dysphonia. Thirdly, multiple hook-wire electrodes can be placed in various sites in and around the larynx for research into the interrelated dynamic processes involved in this intriguing organ. The laryngologist wishing to embark on the first diagnostic initiative is most likely to be rewarded by a cooperative effort with the local neurologist electromyographer.

1.8 NEUROLOGICAL EVALUATION

Some neurological diseases have a clinical profile that includes dysphonia, but the voice disorder is not such that it is a usual first sign. Cerebrovascular diseases (stroke) or degenerative problems such as Parkinson's disease will have phonatory, motor-speech and language components that require specific attention. But others will sometimes present themselves to the otolaryngologist or speech pathologist with the voice disorder being the chief complaint. These may include benign essential tremor and dystonia among others. A full clinical description of these disorders is included in Chapter 3.

Patients with other neurological diseases will and do present to a voice clinic for initial evaluation, so the voice care team may be the first to suspect the presence of amyotrophic lateral sclerosis because of the associated early dysarthria, or early presenting features of multiple sclerosis. Beyond the recognition and facilitation of appropriate referral there is not much further that will be discussed in this chapter.

Needless to say a full neurological examination, particularly of the cranial nerves is essential. For example, tongue muscle fiber fasciculations may be the earliest sign of amyotrophic lateral sclerosis in the head and neck.

1.9 DIAGNOSTIC VOICE THERAPY

Diagnostic or probe therapy seeks to specify the degree and conditions of variability for a patient's dysphonia, and to establish techniques that improve the condition. Results of the probe therapy can be used to estimate prognosis for a voice therapy program. By demonstrating variability in function under controlled conditions, the diagnostic therapy process can be used to modify or eliminate the apparent significance of some organic disease processes. For example, the patient with bilateral nodules and a large posterior glottic chink (PGC) may be trained to reduce the chink magnitude, and demonstrate measurably reduced dysphonia concurrently. In such a case, reduction of muscle misuses contributing to exaggerated PGC becomes the primary management goal, rather than surgical reduction of vocal nodules. In cases where persistent muscle hypertonicity seems to correspond with chronic anxiety states, psychiatric intervention may become the primary management approach, or may be initiated in conjunction with voice therapy. In instances of long-standing muscle misuses that are secondary to psychological or organic pathology, the diagnostic therapy program may consist of several treatment trial sessions to allow for treatment prognosis to be determined. The initial assessment session often does not provide the clinician with adequate time to create an atmosphere of relaxation and trust and to facilitate immediate behavioral or technical changes with patients. Further, a patient's motivation and commitment in the therapy program is not always evident until the clinician can observe his or her response to the therapy program, including cooperation in practising techniques away from the clinic.

1.9.1 Facilitation Techniques for Probe and Symptomatic Therapy

It is important to remember that diagnostic therapy is not by itself a means to confirm psychogenic etiologies for dysphonias, rather it may be supportive of the comprehensive psychological assessment results upon which all psychiatric diagnoses are based. The techniques described below are used in various combinations during diagnostic probe therapy, and the successful ones may be developed further during ongoing voice therapy. Selection of probes depends on the primary clinical features of muscle misuse or vocal impairment demonstrated. When a technique targets correction of a specific sign or symptom, such as 'vocal fold hypoadduction' or 'inappropriately high pitch' it is considered a 'symptomatic technique'. Greater detail on procedural aspects of probe therapy is provided in Chapter 4.

The following is a list of commonly-used facilitation techniques:

- Adduction (forced): pushing; pulling; cough
- Articulation exaggeration; increased orality
- Auditory masking during phonation
- Breathy/flow phonation (increase flow rate)
- Chant (intonation decrease)
- Chewing with phonation
- Character/Impersonation voices
  - imitate opera singer
  - puppet voices
- Distraction: e.g. hum while walking, turning pages, shaking head
- Inhalation phonation
- Intonation increase
- Loudness change
- Lung volume change: e.g. sigh; low-volume /hm/
- Manual manipulation
  - increase thyrohyoid space
  - lower larynx
  - hold tongue forward
  - hold jaw open
- Pitch/register change: e.g. falsetto
- Posture adjustments
  - alter head position
  - supine position
  - lean forward, neck flexed
- Resonance focus adjustment (forward hum/buzz; backed 'covering')
- Simultaneous movements with speech

- head nodding/shaking
- rapid jaw movements /a/
- rapid lip/tongue movements
- Siren imitation
- Speech rate change
- Spontaneous phonation: extend cough; laugh; /mhm/; /hm/
- Tongue position change
- Trills: extend voiced lip or tongue trills
- Voice mode change: singing→speaking; speaking→singing
- Yawn/sigh phonation.

References

1. Akerlund, L., Gramming, P. and Sundberg, J. (1992) Phonetogram and averages of sound pressure levels and fundamental frequencies of speech: comparison between female singers and nonsingers. *Journal of Voice*, **6**(1), 55–63.
2. Awan, N.A. (1991) Phonetographic profiles and f_0-SPL characteristics of untrained versus trained vocal groups. *Journal of Voice*, **5**(1), 41–50.
3. Baer T., Titze I. and Yoshioka H. (1983). Multiple simultaneous measures of vocal fold activity, in *Vocal Fold Physiology: Contemporary Research and Clinical Issues (eds D.M. Bless and J.H. Abbs)*, College-Hill, San Diego, CA.
4. Baken R.J. (1987) *Clinical Measurement of Speech and Voice*, College-Hill, San Diego, CA.
5. Baken R.J. (1992). Electroglottography. *Journal of Voice*, **6**(2), 98–110.
6. Bless D.M., Glaze L.E., Biever-Lowery D.M. *et al.* Stroboscopic, acoustic, aerodynamic and perceptual analysis of voice in normal speaking adults, in *Vocal Fold Physiology*, vol. 5, (ed. R. Baken), Raven Press, New York, NY.
7. Bless D.M., Hirano M. and Feder R.J. (1987) Videostroboscopic evaluation of the larynx. *Ear, Nose and Throat Journal*, **66**(7), 48–58.
8. Bouchayer M., Cornut G., Witzig E. *et al.* (1985) Epidermoid cysts, sulci and mucosal bridges of the true vocal fold: a review of 157 cases. *Laryngoscope*, **95**, 1087–94.
9. Childers D., Naik J., Larar J. *et al.* (1983) Electroglottography, speech, and ultra-high speed cinematography, in *Vocal Fold Physiology: Biomechanics, Acoustics and Phonatory Control* (eds I.R. Titze and R.C. Scherer) Denver Center for the Performing Arts, Denver, CO.
10. Colton R.H. and Casper J.K. (1990) *Understanding Voice Problems*, Williams & Wilkins, Baltimore, MD.
11. Colton R.H. and Conture E.G. (1990) Problems and pitfalls of electroglottography. *Journal of Voice*, **4**(1), 10–24.
12. Damste H. (1970) The phonetogram. *Practica-Oto-Rhino-Laryngologica*, **32**, 185–7.
13. Daniloff R. (1981) Airflow measurements: theory and utility of findings. *Transcripts of the Tenth Symposium on Care of the Professional Voice*, Voice Foundation, New York, NY.
14. Darby J.K. (1981) Speech and voice studies in psychiatric populations, in *Speech Evaluation in Psychiatry*, (ed. J.K. Darby), Grune & Stratton, Inc., New York, NY.
15. Doherty E.T. and Shipp T. (1988) Tape recorder effects on jitter and shimmer extraction. *Journal of Speech and Hearing Research*, **31**, 485–90.
16. Dromey C., Stathopoulos E.T. and Sapienza C.M. (1992) Glottic airflow and electroglottographic measures of vocal function at multiple intensities. *Journal of Voice*, **6**(1), 44–54.
17. Fant G. and Lin Q. (1988) Frequency domain interpretation and derivation of glottic flow parameters. *Speech Transmissions Laboratory – Quarterly Progress and Status Reports*, **2–3**, 1–21.
18. Fritzell B. (1992) Inverse filtering. *Journal of Voice*, **6**(2), 111–14.

19. Garratt B.R., Hanson DG, Berke GS and Precoda (1991) Photoglottography: a clinical synopsis. *Journal of Voice*, **5**(2), 98–105.

20. Gelfer M.-L. (1988) Perceptual attributes of voice: development and use of rating scales. *Journal of Voice*, **2**(4), 320–6.

21. Gramming P. (1991) Vocal loudness and frequency capabilities of the voice. *Journal of Voice*, **5**(2), 144–157.

22. Gramming P., Sundberg J., Ternstrom S. *et al.* (1988) Relationship between changes in voice pitch and loudness. *Journal of Voice*, **2**, 118–26.

23. Hertegard S., Gauffin J. and Karlsson I. (1992) Physiological correlates of the inverse filtered flow waveform. *Journal of Voice*, **6**(3), 224–34.

24. Hirano M. (1981) *Clinical Examination of Voice*, Springer, New York, NY.

25. Isshiki N. (1964) Respiratory mechanism of voice intensity variation. *Journal of Speech and Hearing Research*, **7**, 17–29.

26. Isshiki N. (1965) Vocal intensity and air flow rate. *Folia Phoniatrica*, **17**, 92–104.

27. Iwata S., von Leden H. (1970) Phonation quotient in patients with laryngeal diseases. *Folia Phoniatrica*, **22**, 117–28.

28. Kitzing P. (1985) Stroboscopy-A pertinent laryngological examination. *Journal of Otolaryngology*, **14**(3), 151–7.

29. Klatt D.K. and Klatt L.C. (1990) Analysis, synthesis, and perception of voice quality variations among female and male talkers. *Journal of the Acoustic Society of America*, **87**, 820–57.

30. Komiyama S., Watanabe H. and Ryu S. (1984) Phonographic relationship between pitch and intensity of the human voice. *Folia Phoniatrica*, **36**, 1–7.

31. Koufman J.A., Blalock P.D. (1982) Classification and approach to patients with functional voice disorders. *Annals of Otology, Rhinology and Laryngology*, **91**, 372–7.

32. Laver J. (1980) *The Phonetic Description of Voice Quality*, Cambridge University Press, Cambridge.

33. Laver J. (1991) *Vocal Profiles Analysis*. Queen Margaret College (Edinburgh) and University of Edinburgh Centre for Speech Technology Research, Edinburgh.

34. Lawrence D.H. (1957) *The Oxford Voice*. William Heinemann, London.

35. Lee C.-K. and Childers D.G. (1991) Some acoustical, perceptual, and physiological aspects of vocal quality, in *Vocal Fold Physiology: Acoustic, Perceptual, and Physiological Aspects of Voice Mechanisms* (eds J. Gauffin and B. Hammarberg), Singular San Diego, CA.

36. Lieberman P. (1968) Direct comparison of subglottic and esophageal pressure during speech. *Journal of the Acoustic Society of America*, **43**, 1157.

37. Netsell R., Lotz W.K., DuChane A.S. and Barlow S.M. (1991) Vocal tract aerodynamics during syllable productions: normative data and theoretical implications. *Journal of Voice*, **5**(1), 1–9.

38. Nittrouer S., McGowan R., Milenkovic P. and Beehler D. (1990) Acoustic measurements of men's and women's voices: a study of context effects and covariation. *Journal of Speech and Hearing Research*, **33**, 761–75.

39. Pederson M., Munk E., Moller S. *et al.* (1984) The change of voice during puberty in girls measured with electroglottographic fundamental frequency analysis and phonetograms compared with changes of androgens and secondary sex characteristics. *Acta Otolaryngologica*, (Stockholm), Suppl. **412**, 46–9.

40. Peppard R.C. (1990) Comparison of young adult singers and nonsingers with vocal nodules. *Journal of Voice*, **2**(3), 250–60.

41. Pinto N.B. and Titze I.R. (1990) Unification of perturbation measures in speech signals. *Journal of the Acoustics Society of America*, **87**(3), 1278–89.

42. Ramig L. (1975) Examiner bias in perceptual ratings of nasality in cleft palate speakers. Master's thesis, University of Wisconsin-Madison.

43. Rammage L.A. (1992) Acoustic, aerodynamic and vibratory characteristics of phonation with variable posterior glottis postures. *Doctoral dissertation,* University of Wisconsin-Madison.
44. Rothenberg M. (1992) A multichannel electroglottograph. *Journal of Voice,* **6**(1), 36–43.
45. Rothenberg M. (1973) A new inverse-filtering technique for deriving the glottic air flow waveform during voicing. *Journal of the Acoustic Society of America,* **53**, 1632–45.
46. Rothenberg M. (1977) Measurement of airflow in speech. *Journal of Speech and Hearing Research,* **20**, 155–76.
47. Shoji K., Regenbogen E., Yu J.D. and Blaugrund S.M. (1992) High-frequency power ratio of breathy voice. *Laryngoscope,* **102**, 267–71.
48. Shriberg L.D., Kwiatkowski J. and Rasmussen C. (1990) *Prosody-Voice Screening Profile,* Communication Skill Builders, Tucson, AZ.
49. Smitheran J.R., Hixon T.J. (1981) A clinical method for estimating laryngeal airway resistance during vowel production. *Journal of Speech and Hearing Disorders,* **46**, 138–46.
50. Sodersten M. and Lindestad P.-A. (1992) A comparison of vocal fold closure in rigid telescopic and flexible fiberoptic laryngostroboscopy. *Acta Otolaryngologica,* **112**, 144–50.
51. Sodersten M., Lindestad P.-A., Hammarberg B. (1991) Vocal fold closure, perceived breathiness, and acoustic characteristics in normal adult speakers, in *Vocal Fold Physiology: Acoustic, Perceptual and Physiological Aspects of Voice Mechanisms* (eds J. Gauffin and B. Hammarberg), Singular, San Diego, CA.
52. Spencer L.E. (1988) Speech characteristics of male-to-female transsexuals: a perceptual and acoustic study. *Folia Phoniatrica,* **40**, 31–42.
53. Teitler N. (1992) Examiner bias: influence of patient history on perceptual ratings of videostroboscopy. Master's thesis, University of Wisconsin-Madison.
54. Titze I.R. (1990) Interpretation of the electroglottographic signal. *Journal of Voice,* **4**(1), 1–9.
55. Warren D.W. (1986) Compensatory speech behaviors in cleft palate: A regulation/control phenomenon. *Cleft Palate Journal,* **231**, 251–60.
56. Warren D.W. (1986) Regulation/control of speech aerodynamics *Folia Phoniatrica,* **38**, 368.
57. Yanagasawa E. and Yanagasawa R. (1991) Laryngeal photography. *Otolaryngology Clinics of North America,* **24**(5), 999–1022.
58. Yanigihara N., von Leden H. (1966) Phonation and respiration. Function study in normal subjects. *Folia Phoniatrica,* **18**, 323–40.
59. Yoshioka H., Sawashima M., Hirose H. *et al.* (1977) Clinical evaluation of air usage during phonation. *Japanese Journal of Logopedics and Phoniatrics* **18**, 87–93.

2

Classification of muscle misuse voice disorders

It is apparent that voice disorders frequently labelled 'functional' are associated with laryngeal muscle misuse. This use of the word 'functional' is, however, intrinsically ambiguous, and so we propose an alternative term based on descriptive features of dysfunction: **muscle misuse voice disorders**. Patterns of misuse are traditionally classified by the glottic and supraglottic shapes or postures that are noted on indirect laryngoscopy. A typical example is use of the term **dysphonia plica ventricularis**, when hyperadduction of the false vocal cords is observed in the dysphonic patient. But there are several additional observable forms of misuse.

Persistent phonation with an abnormal laryngeal posture can lead to organic changes such as nodules or polyps, particularly in females with a large posterior glottic chink. We hypothesized that the chink was related to an overall increase in laryngeal muscle tension, and more directly due to inadequate relaxation of the posterior crico-arytenoid muscle during phonation. We employed the term **muscular tension dysphonia** (MTD) to note this condition [16], but it may be that the term **laryngeal isometric** is superior since there are other misuses of the larynx that obviously are manifestations of abnormalities of muscular tension. With this in mind we have evolved a new classification for consideration, based on:

- the laryngeal isometric
- glottic and supraglottic lateral contraction states
- anteroposterior contraction states
- conversion aphonia
- psychogenic bowing
- adolescent transitional dysphonia.

2.1 DEFINITIONS AND RATIONALE

Functional dysphonia is generally used to refer to a voice disorder that is unrelated to identifiable organic disease. This describes a large and diverse group of clinical profiles that collectively imply a disturbance of vocal function due to habituated misuse of voluntary muscles in the oral and pharyngolaryngeal muscle complex, in the breathing system, and in more general postural muscle groups.

Unfortunately, the term 'functional' is still employed by some clinicians to imply an unspecified primary psychological etiology. This is because comprehensive evaluation of a dysphonic patient with a 'normal-looking' larynx that is free of organic disease will often reveal difficulties related both to vocal technique and to psychological distress or conflict. The term 'functional', however, might be employed equally appropriately to refer to aspects of vocal dysfunction that are secondary to organic disease processes. Further, habituated muscle misuse and psychogenic reactions to organic disease frequently interact to produce symptoms that might be broadly categorized under the 'functional' label. Finally, habituated muscle misuse that is psychogenically based or secondary to organic disease can lead to further organic disease processes such as vocal nodules, and in such cases the 'dysfunctional' aspects of a complex etiological profile may be overlooked by those with a reductive bias toward observable organic pathologies. The term 'functional' clearly generates ambiguity in most individual clinical applications.

Dysphonic patients who have structurally normal larynges and demonstrate muscle misuse in the larynx, and those with several interacting causes including habituated muscle tension, are probably better defined as having a 'muscle misuse voice disorder'.

Clearly, the interacting processes that generate voice disorders are not easily defined, nor generalized. This dilemma is reflected in the challenge a clinician faces while attempting to identify and label nonorganic problems. Patients' reports and impressions of events may make the etiological profile even more convoluted, particularly when organic factors, either acute or chronic, existed prior to, or concurrent with, the onset of dysphonia. Commonly occurring organic triggers of muscle misuse voice disorders are upper respiratory tract infections and gastro-esophageal reflux. The task of the voice team is a difficult one: to define and 'sort out' pathological processes that are predisposing, precipitating and perpetuating an individual's dysphonia, and to apply terminology that best describes the relevant ongoing pathophysiological processes for each patient.

The clinician's diagnostic task may be further complicated by signs of organic change secondary to misuse. Vocal nodules are mucosal changes thought to be secondary to vocal abuse and misuse. Nodules often can be identified with a laryngeal mirror and, if assignment of a diagnosis is based solely on this readily identified clinical sign, it seems logical to label the disease process **vocal nodules**. Such an approach to classification, however, focuses on organic pathology, often out of context with the individuals' habitual voice use patterns, and does not allow one to differentiate among the predisposing, precipitating and perpetuating factors involved in the etiology. The consequences for effective management are considerable. In the example of a vocal nodule diagnosis, this label may bias a clinician to focus on the organic change when planning treatment for his or her patients. If instead, the primary etiology (misuse of muscles) is implied in the diagnostic classification, as in the descriptive term **muscular tension dysphonia with acquired vocal nodules**, then management will more likely be directed appropriately, toward reducing chronic dysfunctional muscle use.

A diagnostic classification scheme should be unifying, grouping disorders with common primary causes, yet flexible and expandable, so that individual factors playing etiological roles can be included in descriptions of single patients. The preferred treatment hierarchy may then be implied in a diagnosis. Various authors have attempted to develop classification systems for functional dysphonias that account for some of the issues discussed above. The resultant schemes often have shared common conceptual bases, but different labels. We have attempted to amalgamate a classification system that is comprehensive and promotes the use of diagnostic labels to best reflect all currently recognized patterns of muscle misuse associated with dysphonias. Our long-term goal is a databased descriptive classification scheme that encompasses all etiological factors and facilitates decisions regarding the most efficacious treatment practices.

2.2 PROBLEMS OF CLASSIFICATION

Although clinical patterns described by different authors may bear resemblances, the assumed underlying pathological processes are often different. In addition, the use of terminology is inconsistent. The same term may be used to infer quite different pathological processes, for example, **plica ventricularis, ventricular phonation**, or **ventricular dysphonia** may designate a degree of adducting movement of the ventricular folds simultaneous with adduction of and phonation with the true vocal folds [6]. These terms, however may be employed by others to refer to complete or near complete adduction of, and phonation with, the ventricular folds in the absence of true vocal fold phonation [2]. The latter interpretation seems less often intended, as it represents a fairly rare physiological phenomenon, however the exact phonatory profile is not clear from the label itself. Converse to the situation just described, an apparently similar set of processes may be designated by very different terminology by different authors. **Puberphonia, mutational dysphonia, falsetto phonation** and **adolescent transitional voice disorder** may all refer to a functional dysphonia seen in teenage males who are experiencing difficulty using modal register phonation during or following pubertal growth of the larynx and vocal tract. Commonly, these individuals resort to use of the falsetto register, which may seem to allow for a more stable phonatory pattern, and create a phonatory fundamental frequency that is more familiar. A psychogenic component is often identified in the etiology of this adjustment problem, but is not implied in the diagnostic labels.

Finally, the controversy continues as to the interchangeability of the terms **psychogenic** and **functional** when referring to dysphonias not primarily due to organic pathology. Aronson [2] argues for the use of 'psychogenic' to refer to the broad group of voice disorders that exist in the absence of organic laryngeal pathology. His argument is based on the assumption that 'psychogenic' is broadly synonymous with 'functional' in its application to voice disorder classification, but that it more directly implies an inevitable underlying psycho-emotional disequilibrium. An apparent further motivation for Aronson's dismissal of 'functional' is its semantic breadth, to which he attributes a history of ambiguous interpretations. Brodnitz [5] in employing the term

psychogenic voice disturbances has emphasized the importance of the interaction between organic and psychodynamic factors, which he believes belong together 'like two sides of the coin', in the formation of all 'functional' dysphonias.

Our bias is re-stated here: the terms 'functional' and 'psychogenic' are not synonymous: 'psychogenic' diagnoses should be reserved for those muscle misuse voice disorders that clearly have a primary psycho-emotional etiology, as defined by current standards for psychiatric evaluation [7]. Such a conclusion is not reached solely by exclusion of organic pathogeneses, and often requires a formal psychological evaluation.

2.3 HISTORY OF CLASSIFICATION

Vocal dysfunction has been classified in many ways. A broad distinction was made formerly between **hyperfunctional** and **hypofunctional** voice disorders [8]. Other authors have referred to a diagnostic polarity between **hyperkinesia** and **hypokinesia** [5].

Many authors have agreed that a hyperfunction or hyperkinesia of the laryngeal muscles results in a variety of dysphonia patterns. Further, the secondary organic signs of prolonged misuse of this nature have been highlighted [5, 8, 9, 11, 16]:

- nodules
- polyps
- chronic laryngitis
- contact ulcers
- hypofunction of muscles.

Attempts to classify hypofunctional or hypokinesic voice disorders have resulted in terms such as **paretic hoarseness**, **lateralis paralysis**, **transversus triangle** and **bowing** of the vocal folds [1]. While some authors referred to hypofunctional dysphonia, Jackson [11] employed the term **myasthenia laryngis** to represent the secondary response to hyperfunction, a response he felt accounted for the problems of many professional voice users complaining of voice difficulty. Still other authors have used **phonasthenia** to describe a similar set of signs and symptoms, which were thought to be related to dysfunction of the thyroarytenoid muscles.

In more recent publications, the subclasses 'hyperfunctional' and 'hypofunctional' seem to have yielded to a broader classification of musculoskeletal voice disorders [2, 13, 16, 17].

2.4 MUSCULOSKELETAL APPROACH TO THE CLASSIFICATION OF DYSPHONIAS

Voice disorders can be caused by misuse of the voluntary muscles of phonation including muscles of the larynx, pharynx, jaw, tongue, neck, and respiratory system. General postural misalignment is also common. Some dysphonias can be attributed primarily to incorrect vocal techniques such as:

- poor coordination among respiratory, phonatory, resonatory and articulatory gestures;
- excessive or inadequate laryngeal valving;
- improper resonance focus;
- improper control of pitch and loudness dynamics.

In many cases, extraordinary voice-use demands may contribute to technical incompetence, for example voice use in a chronically noisy environment reduces one's access to auditory feedback, and leads to or intensifies vocal misuse patterns.

Some of the disorders associated with muscular misuses are not associated with observable organic changes to the vocal folds, where others commonly have associated secondary pathologies, including nodules, polypoidal degeneration, chronic laryngitis, or scarring.

In some individuals, muscle misuses may be the direct result of psychological stressors, in which case the resulting dysphonia can legitimately be labelled 'psychogenic'. Psychogenic problems represent failure of an individual to adapt physiologically to a psychological stimulus, usually a conflict-based one [19, 22, 23]. The psychoneuromuscular mechanisms which represent the critical link between emotional conflict and muscular hypertonicity have been well described in the literature of psychosomatic medicine. The overactivity of the autonomic and voluntary nervous systems due to psychological stimuli is related to a variety of neurochemical pressor responses. The voluntary muscles are the final common pathway between the psychological and neurophysiological activities in the formation of somatic symptoms such as dysphonia. Whatmore and Kohli [24] have described a variety of maladaptive disturbance patterns (**dysponeses**) in the signalling system for voluntary muscles which are responses to a variety of psychological states. The dysponetic signals originate in the premotor and motor cortices and influence action potentials in descending pathways, side branches, lower motor neurons, skeletal muscles and the various feedback pathways. Others, including Jacobson [12] and Barlow [3] have also focused on misuse of the voluntary muscles as the final common pathway for psychological conflict and dysfunction. The muscle misuse and misalignment patterns associated with symbolic conversion dysphonias or aphonias lead to severe dysfunction that is primarily psychogenic.

Psychological conflict or distress may be an interacting factor with vocal abuse and misuse in the precipitation and perpetuation of dysphonia, thus contributing to pressor responses in the nervous system which in turn create hypertonicity of the voluntary muscles. Psychological distress may also be secondary to dysphonia, being the direct result of a dysfunctional state. The final result is the same: psychological stimuli lead to inappropriate muscle tone, disturbed feedback, and poor coordination of movements in the final common pathway, the voluntary muscle system [19].

2.4.1 Type 1: Laryngeal Isometric Disorder

The laryngeal isometric pattern is most commonly seen in untrained occupational and professional voice users, including singers, teachers, actors, media personnel, and sales representatives and represents a generalized increase in muscular tension throughout the larynx and paralaryngeal areas. The etiology usually includes a combination of poor vocal technique, extensive and extraordinary voice use demands, and interacting or secondary psychological factors. Anxiety is most commonly identified, and in some cases, the diagnosis of generalized anxiety disorder is made based on criteria listed in the Diagnostic and Statistical Manual of Mental Disorders (DSM-IIIR) [7]. Psychological components may be secondary to dysphonia, rather than a primary etiological factor and this implies a perpetuating influence in sign-symptom formation. In instances where psychological factors clearly play a role in MTD symptom formation we, as voice care clinicians, might do our professions and our patients a great service by adopting a psychosomatic approach to diagnostic classification and treatment of the problem. In psychosomatic medicine, the focus is on social and psychobiological factors that precipitate organic disease. In such a situation, a descriptive diagnosis would reflect the etiological significance of these factors, for example 'anxiety disorder with associated laryngeal isometric dysphonia and bilateral nodules'.

A key feature of the isometric pattern of laryngeal and paralaryngeal hypertonicity relates to the characteristics and role of the posterior crico-arytenoid muscle (PCA) in abducting the glottis. The histological structure of the PCA appears to be well adapted to this role. For example it has more type I muscle fibers than all other intrinsic laryngeal muscles [14]. Thus, when the larynx is in a general hypertonic state, the sustained contraction of the PCA may deflect the arytenoid cartilages down the crico-arytenoid joint and open the posterior commissure, creating a posterior glottic chink (PGC). This hypothesis was supported by a laryngeal muscle pull experiment performed by the authors in 1983 [4]. Dissected fresh human cadaver larynges were held in a frame with the intrinsic muscles attached to strings pulled in the direction of the muscle contraction. It was easily seen that, when the glottis was closed with firm lateral crico-arytenoid and interarytenoid muscle pulls, it took only a light traction on the PCA to open the posterior chink in such a way as to produce a glottic shape such as that seen in this group of patients (Figure 2.1). PGC magnitude also may be associated with hypertonicity in suprahyoid musculature [16].

Studies of clinical populations and normal subjects simulating muscle misuse dysphonias have demonstrated that magnitude of the PGC is directly related to phonatory airflow rate, 'whispery/breathy' perceptions, spectral noise, and distinctive intensity profiles in the acoustic spectra [15–17, 20, 21]. In clinical populations, the laryngeal isometric may be accompanied by other forms of muscle misuse, such as lateral contraction states, which can confound aerodynamic and acoustic profiles.

Disease of the vocal fold mucosa is often identified as a component to the diagnosis, and generally assumed to be secondary to the specific pattern of muscle misuses associated with the laryngeal isometric posture. Hirano [10] has demonstrated the five-layered vocal fold structure in which the superficial two layers, including mucosa and superficial lamina propria (Reinke's space) make up the cover of the vocal fold and the deeper three layers, namely the middle elastic lamina propria, the deep collagenous lamina propria, and the vocalis muscle itself, make up the body of the vocal fold. The muscles contract during phonation, with the strength of the contraction dependent on

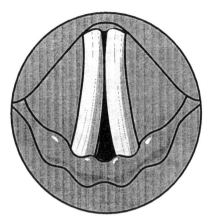

Figure 2.1 The laryngeal isometric. Generalized tension in all the laryngeal muscles is often associated with an open posterior glottic chink due to persistent posterior crico-arytenoid muscle pull during phonation. This leads to secondary mucosal vocal fold changes including nodules, chronic laryngitis, or polypoidal degeneration.

various factors discussed above. During phonation, the cover flows around the leading edge of the vocal fold body, producing the so-called 'mucosal wave' effect seen on stroboscopy. Looseness in the cover overlying the muscle body is necessary for clear phonation. In cases of tense or very loud phonation particularly in the presence of tense vocal folds, shearing stresses can injure the delicate tissue of the superficial lamina propria leading to edema, haemorrhage or fibrosis. These stresses tend to lead to the development of mid-membranous vocal nodules most commonly identified in premenopausal women and prepubertal children. These are also the clinical subgroups that demonstrate the largest PGC magnitudes, and widest interarytenoid spaces relative to vocal fold length. The posterior margin of the nodules corresponds to the anterior margin of the PGC.

This leads one to hypothesize a specific causal relationship between PGC magnitude and bilateral nodules. Perhaps strong adduction forces employed to overcome exaggerated abduction in the posterior glottis lead to greater shearing stresses on the mid-membranous vocal folds at the position where nodules typically develop. Further, lack of adduction posterior to the mid-membranous vocal folds would inhibit development of the mucosal disease there. Subepithelial edema or polypoidal degeneration is the usual form of secondary organic disease found in postmenopausal females, particularly in those who smoke. There is evidence that PGC magnitude and age in women are inversely related [18, 20]. This could provide some explanation for the mucosal disease posterior to the typical nodule site in the older female population. Most adult males will develop a diffuse thickening of the cover that is referred to as 'chronic laryngitis'. Since males have a laryngeal structure that allows for greater closure of the posterior glottis, and indeed PGC magnitudes are generally much smaller in the postpubertal male population, it is not surprising that secondary mucosal disease is more diffuse.

The laryngeal isometric is frequently associated with palpable increases in suprahyoid muscle tension on phonation particularly in higher pitch ranges during singing, and during high vowels and phoneme transitions in connected speech. Elevation of the larynx in the neck and mandible extension may be observed as the patient ascends a sung scale. 'Jaw jut' describes the frequently seen posture that results from simultaneous extension of the neck and mandible.

2.4.2 Type 2: Lateral Contraction

This dysfunctional pattern is a type of tension fatigue syndrome in which the larynx tends to be squeezed or hyperadducted in a side to side direction. It may exist either at the glottic or supraglottic level, or both. The glottic form is usually related to technical errors, and sometimes acute anxiety states may be identified. Supraglottic squeezing, or 'plica ventricularis' on the other hand, is often associated with ongoing psychogenic factors.

Subtype a: Glottic contraction

Simple vocal misuse with hyperadduction of the vocal folds produces a tense-sounding voice due to incorrect vocal technique (Figure 2.2). Phonation is probably associated with high laryngeal resistance forces, which explains why patients complain of 'vocal fatigue' and discomfort at the end of a working day. In some situations the problem is triggered by an organic illness such as an upper respiratory infection, but persistent hoarseness remains many weeks after the viral illness has resolved. Koufman has used the term 'habituated hoarseness' to note this relationship [13].

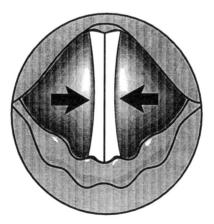

Figure 2.2 Type 2a: Lateral hypercontraction at the glottic level. Frequently seen with generalized postural misuses and tension. May be triggered by an infection or chronic reflux.

The lateral compression in the glottis is generally accompanied by incoordinate breathing such that the larynx functions more like a valve, controlling the rate of expiratory air flow. Proper breath control for speech entails the maintenance of a degree of inspiratory effort during exhalation so that a 'push-pull' mechanism exists in the abdominal and thoracic areas to maintain steady flow of air in the trachea. In this situation, the larynx is not required to function as a flow regulator. When speech-breathing is incoordinate there may be surges of uncontrolled expiratory air, which must then be valved by the glottis during phonation to allow for continued self-oscillation. An effortful and harsh voice results, with rapid fatigue. With ongoing compression, the voice pitch may drop, and vocal fry register may become prominent suggesting that there may be associated anteroposterior constriction. The fatiguing voice may also be accompanied by general fatigue as well as discomfort or pain in the throat.

Laryngoscopy with regular light will generally reveal normal looking structures, although erythema or diffuse thickening of the mucosa may be noted in addition to tight closure of the posterior glottis. Use of the stroboscope will show a prolonged closed phase, reduced vibratory amplitude and suppression of the mucosal wave. Ventricular fold adduction may be seen to a limited degree in association with the glottic level lateral contraction state. In this situation, it is important to differentiate between primary glottic level contraction and primary supraglottic contraction because relegation of a patient to the supraglottic contraction category carries a much stronger inference of psychogenic etiology.

To reiterate, this glottic form of lateral contraction dysphonia is principally a matter of poor vocal habits, posture and technique. The therapy approach is usually directed at correction of the identified phonatory misuses, since specific psychopathological processes are not usually as evident as in subtype b below.

Subtype b: Supraglottic adduction

This pattern tends to predominate in psychogenic dysphonia and can exist either with tightly adducted true vocal folds leading to a high-pitched squeaky voice, or with loose partially abducted vocal folds, in which case the voice is breathy or a tense whisper (Figure 2.3). In the latter situation the tips of the arytenoids are brought together leaving a gap both between the loose membranous cords as well a triangle between the arytenoid bodies. The anterior gap may not be seen because of the adducted ventricular folds which, if almost complete, may only reveal the small whisper-port posteriorly.

When the voice is strident or squeaky it may be difficult to identify whether the sound is generated by:

- the adducted ventricular folds, ie. true false fold phonation;
- tightly adducted true folds obscured by supraglottic structures; or
- the true and false folds functioning together as a unit to create the voice.

The latter two situations are more likely since in most cases the ventricular bands do not adduct fully to the midline.

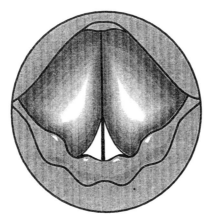

Figure 2.3 Type 2b: Supraglottic lateral contraction, or hyperadduction of the false vocal folds. Tends to be strongly psychologically based.

It has been our experience that the lateral supraglottic squeeze pattern seen on laryngoscopy in patients with a muscle misuse dysphonia is usually associated with unresolved psychological conflict. Conscious or unconscious repression of anger or sadness is common in depressed patients, and primary or secondary gain may be accrued due to presence of the voice disorder. Therapy approaches must combine correction of specific misuses with a careful evaluation and management of the psychological factors. It is in this area that the advantages of a joint approach within a multidisciplinary voice clinic encompassing laryngology, speech pathology, and psychiatry or psychology are most obvious.

2.4.3 Type 3: Anteroposterior Supraglottic Contraction

Koufman has presented a voice type labelled 'Bogart-Bacall' syndrome [13], in which patients exhibit a tension-fatigue dysphonia with phonation at the very bottom of their vocal dynamic ranges. He describes a contraction pattern which results in reduced space between the epiglottis and the arytenoid prominences in the anteroposterior (AP) direction during phonation (Figure 2.4). Individuals using this posture complain of effortful voice and rapid fatigue when speaking at a low pitch but are able to talk more clearly and freely at a higher pitch. This kind of voice can be 'put on' by those wishing to get a particular effect of authority or sultriness, and as a result is often present in the speech of professional voice users. Singers may exhibit a similar AP contraction pattern on phonation in association with tense pharyngolaryngeal postures. This pattern may be used to achieve a particular resonance quality, for example for North American native throat singing, but in other singers it may be unintentional and secondary to technical error. Some singing teachers are beginning to use transnasal flexible videolaryngoscopy with their students to provide instant visual feedback which enables them to avoid this misuse.

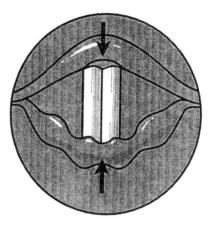

Figure 2.4 Type 3: Anteroposterior supraglottic contraction. A common technical misuse seen in mild, moderate, and severe forms.

This laryngoscopic pattern is not readily seen with mirror examination or with the rigid telescope because the tongue pull may extend the aryepiglottic length. Transnasal examination during connected speech or song is the most effective way to demonstrate this misuse, which may then be subclassified as:

- mild
- moderate
- severe.

2.4.4 Type 4: Conversion Aphonia/Dysphonia

The anxiety that leads to conversion hysteria has produced such mental pain that a physical symptom such as aphonia is much more bearable to the individual [7, 19]. The type of psychological stressors and resulting muscle misuse pattern differs from anxiety related tension misuses associated with type 2a described above. In conversion disorder the misuse may be beyond the awareness of the patient, hence the typical *la belle indifference* facial features. The vocal folds have full movement and can adduct normally for cough or other types of vegetative phonation such as laughter. But they stop short of sufficient adduction for voicing with an attempt to speak (Figure 2.5). Generalized hypertonicity can be identified in the larynx and when sound does come out it is usually high pitched, squeaky, or breathy.

2.4.5 Type 5: Psychogenic Dysphonia with Bowed Vocal Folds

In older patients, presbyphonia is associated with loss of muscular bulk and tone, as well as weakening and fragmentation of elastin and collagen fibers. This so-called 'senile' atrophy is not necessarily the principal factor in patients who are seen to have the

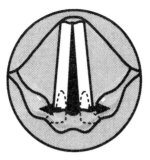

Figure 2.5 Type 4: Conversion aphonia presents a normal larynx in which the vocal folds are held away from the midline during phonation but function well for other duties such as cough.

appearance of bowed vocal folds on indirect laryngoscopy (Figure 2.6). Occasionally, patients who appear to have a psychogenic functional dysphonia will present with a bowed glottis but may resume normal phonation and laryngoscopic appearance after voice and/or psychotherapy. This may also represent one of the forms of dysphonia in 'habituated hoarseness' that follows an upper respiratory tract infection or other organic trigger.

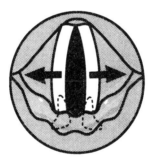

Figure 2.6 Type 5: Psychogenically based dysphonia is not always associated with hyperadduction, and bowing may be seen even when senile atrophy or sulcus vocalis have been excluded.

2.4.6 Type 6: Adolescent Transitional Dysphonia

The normal adolescent voice change during puberty is often accompanied by pitch breaks, register breaks, and a degree of embarrassment. Psychological factors may lead to inhibition of the transitional event and establishment of perpetual falsetto phonation. Laryngoscopy reveals a tense glottis and the cartilaginous glottis may be hyperadducted, restricting phonation to the anterior membranous vocal folds (Figure 2.7). The larynx is generally drawn up tightly into the hyoid bone or base of tongue.

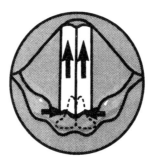

Figure 2.7 Type 6: The voice disorder associated with difficulties making the transition from child to adult male is usually a perpetuated falsetto, and the tension in the posterior glottis is accompanied by a larynx that is held highly and tightly in the neck.

Downward traction on the thyroid cartilages usually results in modal register phonation at a pitch that is more representative of the adult male voice.

Summary

The final common pathway in symptom formation for many dysphonias is misuse of the voluntary muscle systems that are employed for breathing, phonating and resonating. Dysfunctional usage may be the result of a number of interacting factors, and these all need to be taken into account before making final decisions about either classification or therapy.

References

1. Arnold, G.E. (1980) Disorders of laryngeal function, in *Otolaryngology* (eds M.M. Paparella and D.A. Shumrick) W. Saunders Philadelphia, PA., **3**, 2470–88.
2. Aronson, A.E. (1985) *Clinical Voice Disorders: An Interdisciplinary Approach*, 2nd edn, Thieme Medical, New York.
3. Barlow W. (1973). *The Alexander Principle*, Victor Gollanz, London.
4. Belisle G. and Morrison M.D. (1983) Anatomic correlation for muscle tension dysphonia. *Journal of Otolaryngology*, **12**, 319–21.
5. Brodnitz F.S. (1959) Vocal rehabilitation. *American Academy of Ophthalmology and Otolaryngology Monograph*, Whiting, Rochester, NY.
6. Colton R.H. and Casper J.K. (1990) *Understanding Voice Problems. A Physiological Perspective for Diagnosis and Treatment.* Williams & Wilkins, Baltimore, MD.
7. *Diagnostic and Statistical Manual of Mental Disorders*, 3rd Edn – Revised (DSM-III-R) (1987), American Psychiatric Association, Washington, DC.
8. Froeschels E. (1943) Hygiene of the voice. *Archives of Otolaryngology* **37**, 122–30.
9. Greene M.C.L. (1972) *The Voice and its Disorders*, J.B. Lippincott, Philadelphia, PA.
10. Hirano M. (1974) Morphological structure of the vocal cord as a vibrator and its variations. *Folia Phoniatrica*, **26**, 89–94.
11. Jackson C. (1940) Myasthenia laryngis. *Archives of otolaryngology* **32**, 434–63.
12. Jacobson E. (1970) *Modern Treatment of Tense Patients*, Charles C. Thomas, Springfield, IL.

13. Koufman J.A. and Blalock P.D. (1982) Classification and approach to patients with functional voice disorders. *Annals of Otology, Rhinology and Laryngology*, **91**, 372–7.
14. Malmgren L., Gacek R. and Etzler C. (1983) Muscle fibre types in the human posterior crico-arytenoid muscle: a correlated histochemical and ultrastructural morphometric study, in *Vocal Fold Physiology: Biomechanics, Acoustics and Phonatory Control* (eds I.R. Titze and R.C. Sherer). Denver Center for the Performing Arts, Denver, Co, pp. 41–56.
15. Milenkovic P., Bless D.M. and Rammage L.A. (1991) Acoustic and perceptual characterization of vocal nodules, in *Vocal Fold Physiology: Acoustic, Perceptual, and Physiological Aspects of Voice Mechanisms* (eds J. Gauffin and B. Hammarberg), Singular San Diego, CA, pp. 265–72.
16. Morrison M.D., Rammage L.A., Belisle G.M. *et al.* (1983) Muscular tension dysphonia. *Journal of Otolaryngology*, **12**, 302–6.
17. Morrison M.D., Nichol H. and Rammage L.A. (1986) Diagnostic criteria in functional dysphonia. *Laryngoscope*, **96**, 1–8.
18. Peppard R.C. (1990) Effects of selected vocal characteristics of female singers and non-singers. Doctoral dissertation, University of Wisconsin-Madison.
19. Rammage L.A., Nichol H. and Morrison M.D. (1987) The psychopathology of voice disorders. *Human Communication Canada*, **11**, 21–25.
20. Rammage L.A. (1992) Acoustic, aerodynamic and vibratory characteristics of phonation with variable posterior glottis postures. Doctoral dissertation, University of Wisconsin-Madison.
21. Rammage L.A., Peppard R.C. and Bless D.M. (1989) Aerodynamic, laryngoscopic and perceptual–acoustic characteristics in dysphonic females with posterior glottal chinks: a retrospective study. *Journal of Voice (New York)*, **6**, 64–78.
22. Selye H. (1976) *The Stress of Life*, McGraw-Hill, New York, NY.
23. Stoyva J. (1978) Why should muscular relaxation be clinically useful? Some data and $2\frac{1}{2}$ models. A psychophysiological model of stress disorders as a rationale for biofeedback training, in (ed) *Proceedings of the Second Meeting of the American Association for the Advancement of Tension Control* (ed. F.J. McGuigan), University of Chicago, Chicago, IL.
24. Whatmore G.B. and Kohli D.R. (1974) The physiopathology and treatment of functional disorders. Grune & Stratton, New York, NY.

3

Medical aspects of voice disorders

Optimal medical management of a patient with a voice disorder requires accurate diagnosis. When hoarseness is accompanied by a clearly identifiable acute upper respiratory tract infection, or follows excessive shouting at an athletic event, the diagnosis may be easy, but in other situations the cause and best treatment may be more elusive.

When visited by a patient who is hoarse, the physician may wish to use a decision tree (Figure 3.1).

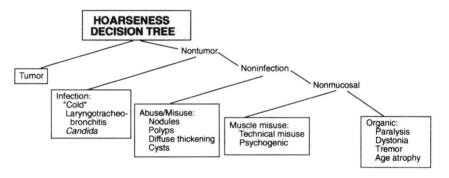

Figure 3.1 A 'decision tree' schema to assist in the evaluation of hoarseness.

This decision tree allows the evaluator to work through a list of potential diagnosis groups in an orderly fashion, and is a useful thought process to follow. We will follow it through this chapter.

3.1 TUMORS

Tumors tend to produce an indolent, slowly progressive hoarseness and patients who are hoarse worry about cancer. In reality, the assurance that there is no cancer present may be all that the patient needs or wants.

Laryngeal tumors may be benign or malignant. A full discussion of this topic is well beyond the scope of this book and the reader wishing more detail should refer to one of the many current references on this topic, but a few general comments are in order.

Laryngeal papilloma is a benign, warty growth which is more common in children than in adults and is linked to the human papilloma virus. It is thought that the larynx becomes infected during birth, and treatment generally consists of repeated laryngoscopic laser excision. This is discussed in more detail in Chapter 7.

The most common malignant tumor in the larynx is squamous cell carcinoma affecting the glottis. The typical patient with cancer of the vocal fold is a male in his 60s or 70s with a harsh raspy or breathy voice that came on insidiously. He is almost always a long-time smoker. When laryngeal cancer is suspected, referral to an otolaryngologist is essential. Squamous cell carcinoma can be diffuse or localized, keratotic or erythematous, exophytic or ulcerative, appear hard or soft, and may confuse the examiner's eye. A high index of suspicion is needed.

Airway obstruction or neck nodal metastases are not usually associated with early glottic cancer, but may develop if the disease is allowed to progress. When neck nodes or airway obstruction accompany the early presenting features, the primary tumor may have started in the supraglottic larynx or hypopharynx, where it can reach a considerable size before symptoms develop. Most early vocal fold cancers can be treated effectively with radiation therapy or limited surgery, both of which result in high cure rates. T1 lesions (confined to the glottis and with normal mobility) can be controlled in over 90% of patients, but curability of late lesions drops dramatically and treatment may involve total laryngectomy.

3.2 INFECTION

Inflammation of the larynx, with redness and swelling of the mucosal membranes, commonly accompanies an upper respiratory tract infection. There are three main groups of viral infection in the upper aerodigestive tract.

- The common cold viruses principally cause inflammation in the lining of the nose and sinuses and, in most cases, the degree of actual laryngitis is slight, but the common cold is occasionally accompanied by laryngeal edema and consequent hoarseness.
- Adenoviruses are the usual culprit in cases of severe sore throat, accompanied by fever, pain on swallowing, tender lymph nodes in the neck, and swollen, red tonsils. As with the common cold, while there may be mild hoarseness, communication is not usually impaired.
- The organisms that cause laryngo-tracheo-bronchitis are often the influenza, or para-influenza, viruses. This is the illness that produces the most severe voice change and sudden curtailment of vocal performance.

In children the laryngeal edema leads to narrowing of the airway just below the vocal folds, resulting in inspiratory stridor, or 'croup'. Although a similar severity of inflammation occurs in adults, the larynx is big enough to avoid obstruction, but the hoarseness, cough, and general misery can be intense. This common illness results in a low pitched, hoarse voice with pitch or phonation breaks or even aphonia. Physical examination shows a thickened, reddened tracheal and subglottic mucosa, and the inflammatory changes here may be easier to see than in the vocal folds themselves. This adult variant of the childhood type of laryngotracheitis is probably the most common cause of voice loss due to 'laryngitis'.

Dysphonia associated with these illnesses is temporary and not a major problem unless the patient happens to be a professional voice user, such as a singer. Rest and extra hydration are the mainstays of treatment. But an urgent need for voice, as for a major concert, may lead to an array of treatment options up to systemic steroids with antibiotic coverage.

Case 1

Sandra Soprano is a 39-year-old diva who had the leading role in a local production of *La Boheme*. On the day prior to the third of her four performances, she developed a tickle in her throat and a minor but irritating cough. She felt generally tired and yet the demands of the performance gave her the energy to carry on. She managed to get through the role reasonably well, although some of her high notes were effortful and the next morning, she felt generally unwell. The pitch of her speaking voice had dropped a tone and her throat was slightly sore. On examination the nose, oral cavity and pharynx were normal, but indirect laryngoscopy showed slightly pink and glistening vocal folds. Since the examiner had not seen this patient before, it was hard to say whether the examination was revealing features within the bounds of what might be considered normal for this individual. Of greatest concern, however, was a distinctly thickened and irritated tracheal mucosa visible between the vocal folds, and thus the diagnosis of a laryngotracheitis, likely of viral cause, was entertained.

Without further vocal demands the treatment of this situation is very easy and consists of adequate hydration and rest but, in two days, Sandra was scheduled to sing again to a sold-out house of 3000 opera fans. The understudy was poorly prepared, but could sing the part from the wings leaving Sandra to walk through the staging. Sandra had no singing commitments for three weeks after this show (an important point) and wanted to carry on if at all feasible. It was therefore decided to reduce the inflammation as much as possible and, coupled with rest, fluids, and the risk of injury, allow Sandra to carry on.

Treatment was started using prednisone 30 mg twice daily, plus amoxicillin 250 mg eight-hourly, to reduce the chance of opportunistic bacterial infections. Her usual good hydration habits were supplemented with steam inhalations and a topical beclomethasone spray. The prednisone dosage was planned to taper off over 10 days. Guaifenesin (guaiphenesin) was also used to thin secretions.

The following day Sandra's speaking voice pitch seemed more normal and she was feeling a little better although, as is usual in this situation, she felt a little 'strange'. By performance day the adrenalin rush, coupled with an extra careful and lengthy warm up carried her through.

This scenario is not terribly uncommon, but in some instances the laryngologist together with the singer must decide that to attempt such a 'rescue' is not worth the risk. The degree of laryngotracheitis and the early response to treatment will help make this decision.

Bacterial infection may occur primarily or be secondary to a viral illness. The erythema tends to be more severe and accompanied by pain and fever. There may be thicker purulent discharge or ulceration. Bacterial infection with pathogens such as *Streptococcus* or *Staphylococcus* may produce subglottic thickening and some airway narrowing as well as severe hoarseness. Supraglottitis due to *Hemophilus influenzae* can lead to a major airway emergency and consideration in a text about voice disorders is inappropriate.

Tuberculosis can rarely affect the larynx, usually secondarily to a pulmonary infection. Examination usually reveals what appear to be fairly smooth subepithelial pale nodules variably located around the supraglottic larynx.

Fungal infection of the larynx is actually quite common. The usual cause is *Monilia* introduced by regular use of corticosteroid inhalers, particularly in the presence of diabetes of immunological abnormalities. Numerous white flecks of *Candida* colonies usually scatter themselves around the arytenoid areas, aryepiglottic folds and epiglottis. Thicker, white, keratotic-looking plaques may occur on the vocal folds themselves and be mistaken for dysplastic or malignant lesions. The association with surrounding typical monilial colonies is the giveaway, and the fact that the vocal fold lesions will disappear with antifungal therapy. A treatment that is effective in most cases is nystatin (Mycostatin) tablets dissolved slowly in the mouth three times daily. The oral suspension used as a gargle does not seem to work as well, probably because it is washed away so quickly.

3.3 CHRONIC NONINFECTIVE LARYNGITIS

With infection excluded, the decision tree passes on to noninfective mucous membrane changes of the vocal folds. Chronic inflammatory changes in the glottis can be produced by smoking, allergy, gastro-esophageal reflux disease, or voice abuse. The changes in the lining of the vocal fold may vary from a thickening at the middle portion of the vibrating vocal fold that may be termed nodules or polyps, depending on the physical appearance and relative thickness of the epithelium itself, to changes in underlying connective tissue.

Diffusely thickened vocal fold mucosa, caused by persistent chronic irritation such as cigarette smoke, may be further accompanied by keratosis or **leukoplakia**, meaning white plaques. In this situation the irritative processes lead to a disruption of the normal maturation processes through the levels of the epithelial lining, and may have malignant potential. This not to imply that nodules resulting from chronic voice abuse in a singer or in a child with 'screamer's nodules' have any chance of becoming a cancer, but it illustrates the wide range of causes and pathologic processes that may lead to glottic mucosal thickening and resultant hoarseness.

This change is a general indication for surgery, with the usual procedure being laser ablation of the thick white tissue, down to the middle layer of laminal propria. Postoperatively the mucous membrane regenerates with a more normal appearance, but the mucosal wave on stroboscopy can be inhibited by scarring and a degree of huskiness of the voice may persist.

Gastro-esophageal reflux disease is an organic cause of chronic laryngitis and voice misuse that can be identified and managed effectively. In the presence of reflux, even when it is mild, there often is increased pharyngo-esophageal muscle tone, and accompanying symptoms include postnasal drip, a lump in the throat, and the feeling of a need to clear the throat (which is usually acted upon frequently by the sufferer and therefore contributes to further vocal abuse and awareness). In addition, the muscles of the pharynx and larynx tend to be tense, which promotes misuse and can contribute to wear-and-tear injury in the larynx. Following the general principles of antireflux therapy can be of significant help [8]. The antireflux instruction sheet that we use as a handout for patients is provided in Appendix A.

Although seasonal allergies may cause hoarseness similar to that accompanying a cold, it is surprising that this is not a common problem. Even in patients with significant nasal allergies or asthma, the incidence of voice problems is low. The severity of other allergic accompaniments should help identify which patients are suffering dysphonia of allergic cause.

Repeated vomiting associated with bulimia nervosa can also produce chronic laryngitis, and this possibility should be borne in mind in hoarse adolescent females [7].

Case 2
   Beryl Belcher, aged 28 years, has been trying to get going on a pop singing career but on a number of occasions she has suddenly lost her voice following an evening of effortful singing. Examination shortly after one of these episodes revealed that she had a diffuse subepithelial haemorrhage along the entire length of the right vocal fold. Total voice rest was recommended and the hematoma resolved leaving only a bright red nodular mass on the superior surface of the cord, consistent with the diagnosis of a capillary hemangioma (Figure 3.2a).

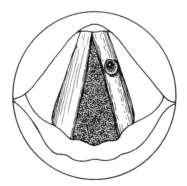

Figure 3.2a A bright red microhemangioma is noted on the superior surface of the right vocal fold, as seen in case 2.

Since it has been shown that vocal fold telangiectasis and microhemangiomata are often associated with the repeated vomiting of bulimia nervosa the subject was broached and it was determined that the patient had in fact been bulimic between the ages of 16 and 18. Careful laser ablation of the vascular anomaly stopped the occurrences of bleeding.

3.4 MISUSE AND ABUSE

This topic is covered extensively elsewhere in this book, but a few comments will be included here to help us follow along the decision tree. Misuse and abuse of the voice are common causes of chronic inflammatory changes in the larynx in the absence of infection.

Case 3

Betty Belter, aged 23 years, has always been called upon for the lead roles in the school or community theatre. She is outgoing, attractive, and has a natural pleasing singing voice and musicality. She is socially active, enjoying the company of others in nightclubs on the weekend, where she also works as a hostess to help augment her daytime salary. Betty's regular work as a receptionist is vocally demanding and she is frequently hoarse by the end of a stressful working day. She smokes a pack of cigarettes a day, as does her boyfriend. Incidentally, the relationship with her boyfriend seems to be coming apart.

Betty was encouraged to become involved with a rock band that a group of friends were starting up. She would, of course, be the lead singer. She has now lost much of her upper vocal register and is concerned about the degree of breathiness in her voice that remains even after a few days of rest. Singing lessons have been suggested but her friends say that they would only ruin her 'naturally good' voice.

The fleshy, sessile, almost polypoid nodules seen in Betty's larynx reflect her characteristic isometric muscle misuse, combined with voice abuse and cigarette smoking (Figure 3.2b). Primary management of this problem requires help with behavioral modification through counselling, direct voice therapy and cessation of smoking. Should it become necessary to consider 'trimming' the vocal nodules, the procedure should be in combination with the primary treatments, and consist of a conservative reduction of polypoid tissue while retaining as full a mucosal cover as possible. A more widespread 'stripping' would result in the problem illustrated in case 4.

Misuse and abuse of the voice can result in wear and tear on the vocal folds and development of epithelial thickening, referred to as vocal nodules, polyps, or chronic laryngitis. The term 'misuse' implies that the vocal technique is faulty and the true vocal folds, which are made up of voluntary muscle, are forced to vibrate under undue stress and tension. In order to produce a clear, effortless tone, the vocal folds must be adducted without too much force, so that expiratory flow can serve to sustain vibration, rather than force apart a tightly closed valve. A common misuse involves tight glottic

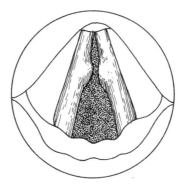

Figure 3.2b Soft sessile vocal nodules characteristic of case 3.

adduction and forceful expiration, leading to muscle fatigue as well as inflammation producing shearing stresses on the vocal folds.

Voice abuse refers to exuberant overuse of the voice from such activities as excessive singing, loud talking (especially in noisy places), shouting, cheering, etc. People who abuse their voices often tend to have a problem with muscle misuse as well, and the cumulative effects can be exponential. Vocal fold changes occur more rapidly with vocal abuse in such individuals, compared to those whose habitual vocal technique is more 'correct'. Counselling about voice use, coupled with direct voice therapy with or without singing lessons, can be an essential part of the retraining required to manage this problem. Vocal nodules may be a sign of the misuse and abuse problem rather than being the primary problem, and their presence does not necessarily mean they should be removed. If the misuse and abuse are controlled, nodules often resolve. Even if they remain, the patient's voice problems may resolve and the presence of nodules may cease to be an issue.

3.5 LARYNGEAL TRAUMA

Although external trauma to the larynx, such as may occur in a motor vehicle accident, can result in disorganization or scarring and produce voice alterations, it is relatively uncommon and usually does not present a diagnostic dilemma. But internal trauma to the vocal folds from surgical treatment or intubation is more frequent and often can be overlooked. Although direct injury to vocal folds at the time of intubation for a surgical procedure is extremely unusual, its effects can be devastating, particularly if the patient earns a living by voice use. Physicians who are planning to pass an endotracheal tube in a patient who is a singer or professional speaker should discuss this possibility with the patient beforehand, use the smallest tube that is sufficient for adequate ventilation, and take available measures to prevent injury. Injury may occur from subluxation of the crico-arytenoid joint if the tip of an endotracheal tube catches in the laryngeal ventricle and then is pushed against this resistance. When this does occur, it tends to be in a situation in which the intubation is a life-saving measure, and a subsequent voice problem is not high on the list of concerns.

Another major cause of internal laryngeal injury is excessive removal of mucosa or glottic tissue at the time of surgical treatment of disease, whether it be benign or malignant. It was relatively common in the past to see well-healed, white vocal folds in a woman still complaining bitterly about a harsh, squeaky voice several months after a surgical stripping of glottic mucosa. The speech pathologist may have been left to struggle along with the patient and sometimes a better voice finally returned. Any resultant scar on the vocal fold can inhibit normal vibration and leave the patient with an unpleasant dysphonic voice. Stroboscopic examination now readily shows us the damage that was being done and how re-epithelialization was accompanied by tethering of the mucosa to the deeper tissues and stiffening of the fold through scar formation. Happily, surgical techniques have changed so that, with mucosa sparing procedures, this is a less common problem. Of course it is an expected and accepted side effect of endoscopic tumor removal.

Case 4

'Gravel Gerty' Green arranged a visit to her doctor because she became tired of being called 'sir' on the telephone. Her church choir leader suggested that she move from the alto to the tenor section. She wanted to know if there was anything that could be done to raise the pitch of her voice back to its previous level. Consequently a laryngoscopy and removal of edematous vocal fold mucosa was performed. Four months later her voice had not yet recovered, remaining squeaky, strained, and breathy in spite of a number of voice therapy sessions postoperatively.

Stroboscopic videolaryngoscopy showed that both vocal folds were stiff, and the mucosal wave dampened, more severely on the right side than the left. There appeared to be an area towards the anterior end of the fold that lacked bulk and also was much less pliable on strobe exam (Figure 3.2c).

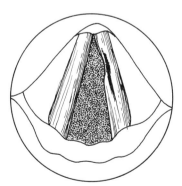

Figure 3.2c A stiff indented scar is noted on the anterior half of the right vocal fold of case 4. This is the result of tethering of mucosa following a stripping of polypoidal disease.

As was demonstrated in Gerty's case, when vocal fold stripping leaves wide areas bare, the regenerating glottic mucosa may become densely adherent to the underlying lamina propria, and simply not vibrate well. It may slowly soften with time but persistent dysphonia is difficult to treat. Submucosal injections of collagen have been shown to be helpful in some cases [5].

Subepithelial hemorrhage of the vocal fold is an infrequent but very important and serious event that can put a singing career on hold. It may be prevented by microlaser vaporization of any small hemangiomata or telangiectatic vessels, particularly in a singer who has already had one bleed. After a bleed, of course, a period of absolute voice rest is essential, and if the hematoma is at all bulky then it should probably be evacuated surgically.

3.6 OTHER MUCOSAL DISEASES

3.6.1 Contact Ulcer and Granuloma

Contact ulcers and granulomas in the larynx are inflammatory lesions that occur over the vocal processes and medial surface of the arytenoids in the posterior larynx. They usually are unilateral but bilateral lesions have also been seen. In the typical case, the contact granuloma occurs in someone who is suffering from gastro-esophageal reflux disease and has a habitually aggressive style of voice use. A common variety of this disorder is the true post-intubation granuloma, which is usually bilateral. Management of contact granulomas may entail biopsy early in the course of treatment, but generally centres on reflux management and close follow-up, since under this therapy the granulomas may resolve spontaneously.

Case 5

Larry Litigator spends much of his day in the courtroom. He loves his work. He also loves black coffee and late, Mexican dinners. His co-workers have begun to complain about his constant throat clearing, and he finds that the amount of effort to keep talking all day has greatly increased.

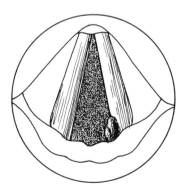

Figure 3.2d Contact granuloma over the right vocal process, as seen in case 5.

The most obvious sign seen on laryngoscopic examination is a heaped up granular lesion overlying the medial surface of the right arytenoid cartilage (Figure 3.2d). The vocal folds look normal but stroboscopic assessment demonstrates excessive medial compression, evidenced by a prolonged closed phase of the vibratory cycle. As in Larry's case, **contact granulomata** are frequently associated with chronic gastro-esophageal reflux, together with a muscle misuse voice disorder. Antireflux management as described above and in Appendix A. together with ranitidine 150 mg twice daily results in a slow resolution of the granuloma. Larry also attends a group voice therapy program that targets the needs of professional speakers, and has been very gratified by his increased ability to perform in court.

3.6.2 Cysts, Sulci, and Mucosal Bridges

Other mucosal changes that are not directly related to voice misuse and abuse, such as intracordal cysts and vocal fold sulci are seen occasionally, and were not well recognized until our ability to examine that larynx was enhanced by video magnification and stroboscopic study of vocal fold vibration. Bouchayer *et al.* [3] described these lesions as representing a spectrum of disorders related to embryological development. Hypothetically cysts are due to a failure of development that leaves a remnant of mucosa in Reinke's space below the 'normal' mucosal cover. This then can lead to a cyst in Reinke's space that contains a white, mucoid substance and has a very delicate mucosal lining. The overlying vocal fold mucosa is usually loosely adherent, but the cyst is densely stuck to the underlying lamina propria (Figure 3.2e). Special sets of microlaryngeal surgical instruments have been developed to permit cysts to be delicately dissected free. An incision is made along the superior surface of the vocal fold, in the direction of the fold, just through the mucous membrane which is then elevated medially towards the free edge of the vocal fold exposing the cyst. Since the deep aspect of the cyst is very adherent to the laminal propria below it, great care must be taken to peel it away without breakage. If the cyst does rupture then the surgeon must decide whether to try to remove all of the cyst lining with some surrounding fibrous tissue or to stop the surgery and come back to try another day after the cyst has re-formed.

The lesion can also be open to the laryngeal lumen as a sinus or **sulcus vocalis**. An overlying flap of mucous membrane may be present that makes the sulcus difficult to see even with videostroboscopy or, more commonly, only the densely stuck deep part exists and this is more obvious as a groove along the free edge of the fold (Figure 3.2f). Stroboscopic exam clearly shows the sulcus as being tethered to the underlying vocal ligament. In regular light the folds look bowed. In Western Canada, this lesion seems to be prevalent in the population from the Indian subcontinent.

Surgical treatment of vocal fold sulci in which a strip of mucosa is very densely adherent to the free edge of the fold, is difficult and several less-than-satisfactory techniques have been tried and discarded.

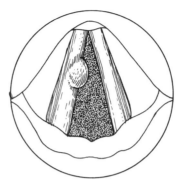

Figure 3.2e Intracordal cyst of the left vocal fold.

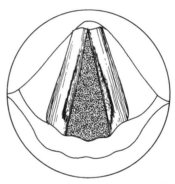

Figure 3.2f Sulcus vocalis. The mucosa is densely adherent to the fibrous layers of the lamina propria, and does not vibrate well.

3.6.3 Congenital Web

Large webs are obvious and produce significant degrees of hoarseness. They occur in the anterior commissure and while they may often look simple and thin, the thinness is usually only found at the posterior free margin of the web. Most anteriorly they splay superiorly and inferiorly into quite a thick base that includes a firm fibrous core. This makes what should seem to be an easy endoscopic division likely to fail, and necessitates special procedures for successful ablation. However the mucosal microweb which, until the advent of video stroboscopic examination techniques, was not seen or deemed important, may produce a subtle loss of vocal power and can be dealt with by a simple snip.

3.6.4 Crico-arytenoid Joint Problems

The synovial crico-arytenoid joints are subject to the same arthritic problems as other joints although involvement is remarkably uncommon in rheumatoid disease. Most joint mobility difficulties are related to intubation trauma, from prolonged intubation or acute injury producing subluxation. The subluxed arytenoid can be seen to be asymmetrically positioned, and the vocal process is generally more anterior and inferior to the normal side. The vocal fold itself appears shorter and thicker, and may look bowed.

Chronic gastro-esophageal reflux disease can also promote periarticular inflammation and fibrosis that can stiffen the joint and limit mobility. Laryngological examination will reveal erythema of the posterior glottis and limited excursion, with or without ulceration or granulation tissue medial to the arytenoid cartilage.

3.7 PSYCHOGENIC MUSCLE MISUSE DYSPHONIA

Returning to our decision tree, we note that in some hoarse patients an examination of the larynx reveals it to be structurally and mucosally normal, without any evidence of tumor, infection, or any of the disorders described above. Patients who are heavy voice users, often with income-related vocal activity, may have hoarseness directly related to laryngeal muscle tension, even though it has not yet caused mucosal changes. The management of these patients is covered extensively in Chapter 4.

Sometimes, however, the cause of the disorder is primarily psychogenic. In these patients the voice may vary from almost normal to a whisper, and phonation attempts may be characterized predominantly by glottic fry, laryngeal effort, or high-pitched squeaky sounds. Various psychopathological processes can contribute to dysphonia, as outlined in detail in Chapter 1 and Chapter 5.

Medical 'treatment' may be largely to reassure the patient about the absence of organic diseases, and to begin to pave the way towards effective resolution of the problem by way of collaborative referral to those providing voice and psychotherapy.

3.8 NEUROGENIC VOICE DISORDERS

3.8.1 Vocal Fold Paralysis

Vocal fold paralysis is the most common neurogenic voice disorder. A unilateral recurrent laryngeal nerve paralysis may result in a spectrum of problems, from a weak breathy voice to aspiration and difficulties with cough. Immediately after onset the paralysed vocal fold may be too far lateral from the midline to permit approximation by the mobile fold. As a result the voice may be weak and breathy. Occasionally, a double tone, referred to as diplophonia, may be heard. In many patients with unilateral recurrent laryngeal nerve paralysis, recovery of the voice occurs either through a mechanism of spontaneous medialization, without the return of full mobility, or with full recovery. The medialization may be due to random re-innervation of the endolaryngeal muscles, with resultant improvement in muscular tone. When this occurs, the voice may be normal.

The main indication for surgical treatment of vocal fold paralysis is ineffective cough and aspiration, but restitution of voice may also be a reason for surgical intervention. A common surgical technique is to inject teflon (or sometimes Gelfoam) into the tissues lateral to the paralysed vocal fold. This technique was originally introduced by Arnold in 1962 [1]. Other forms of surgery include medialization through external placement of a laryngeal implant, or selective muscle re-innervation.

There are advantages and disadvantages for each of the surgical methods of voice augmentation for unilateral recurrent laryngeal nerve paralysis. There is no one best method, and each clinical situation must be considered on its own merits.

Augmentation by teflon injection has stood the test of time, and may be done in the operating room via direct laryngoscopy, or in the clinic indirectly or transcutaneously. There is a consensus that the voice results may not be as good in the long term as with other techniques, but this treatment still has great value, particularly for quick rehabilitation of patients with mediastinal metastatic carcinoma.

Isshiki, Okamura and Ishikawa [6] have described two types of **thyroplasty** that are very effective in rehabilitating vocal paralysis. Vocal fold medialization can be achieved via an external neck incision and sub-perichondrial insertion of a silastic block prosthesis through a window cut into the thyroid cartilage. This medializes the cord in much the same way as teflon adds bulk to the deep laryngeal tissues, but without the associated stiffness or inflammation. It also is reversible or 'tuneable' in that the prosthesis may be removed or exchanged for one of another size.

They have also described a technique for arytenoid adduction that involves attaching a suture on the muscular process of the arytenoid and passing it forward to an anchor point in the anterior thyroid cartilage. Suture tension can be adjusted to stretch and medialize the vocal fold. While more difficult to perform, this technique gives excellent voice results in selected cases.

Neuromuscular re-innervation procedures are still in the evaluative phase, but the hypothesis is that re-innervated muscle will have bulk and tone and may vibrate more effectively, and with a restored mucosal wave. A nerve crossover procedure between the ansa cervicalis and the recurrent nerve, as described by Crumley, Izdebski and McMicken [4], may be the best way to do this. An example ideal patient is one that has lost the recurrent nerve in the chest due to aortic arch surgery.

3.8.2 Dystonia and Tremor

The term **spastic** or **spasmodic dysphonia** (SD) implies that a patient with a normal-looking larynx at rest, has a strained, often dysfluent voice. It is usually insidious in onset and progresses over months or years. This disorder may be related to stress or psychological factors, but recently many patients are being identified as having a focal dystonia akin to blepharospasm or writer's cramp. Effective management of SD patients requires a team approach including the contributions of an otolaryngologist, speech pathologist, neurologist, and psychiatrist.

Not unusually, the larynx of a patient suffering from idiopathic adductor spasmodic dysphonia will look normal, at least with regular light. Stroboscopic exam will reveal the increased closed phase that is typical of a laryngeal dystonia. The excursion of the mucosal wave will also be reduced. There is a better chance that the voice and glottic appearance on phonation will be more normal at high pitch where less of the bulk of the vocalis muscle has to be involved with the vibratory cycle, and adductive tension may be lower. Low pitched phonation will more likely be spasmodic, even on indirect examination where the tongue is being forcefully extended. Hyperadducted supraglottic structures may be associated with dystonia.

The term **dystonia** refers to the situation where a muscle or group of muscles becomes involuntarily hypertonic, and the resultant spasm results in its inability to function normally. Typical examples around the head and neck include cervical dystonia (spasmodic torticollis), blepharospasm, Meige's syndrome (blepharospasm plus oromandibular dystonia), as well as the now commonly recognized spasmodic dysphonia. Not all spasmodic dysphonia symptoms can be definitely attributed to this central neuromuscular processing disorder, since some patients have an identical spasmodic voice ailment which has been shown to have an entirely psychological cause. Still, being able to identify previously puzzling voice-disordered patients as having a focal dystonia relieves much frustration for the sufferer and therapist alike. The ability to render near-miraculous resolution of the symptoms using botulinum toxin makes life more pleasant for patients and voice care teams. As mentioned above, spasmodic dysphonia is sometimes confused with tremor as implied in the subclassification list below.

Dystonic adductor spasm of the larynx can also produce difficulties with respiration and the patient with adductor breathing dystonia will usually come to the otolaryngologist with an airway complaint rather than being so concerned with the voice, but that does not mean that the voice aspects are not present. Fortunately these patients may also respond to botulinum toxin, but many still need airway support via a tracheotomy. The psychiatric interactions in this disorder are probably quite active but confusing, with the chicken–egg dilemma being operant.

Focal dystonia may rarely affect other muscles in the larynx. Posterior crico-arytenoid involvement may lead to abductor vocal spasm that produces an inconsistently weak, breathy, and dysfluent voice, and the clinical picture may be confused with a more common psychogenic hypoadducting dysphonia not unlike that seen in many cases of so-called hysterical aphonia. But true abductor dystonia appears to exist and may respond well to injection of botulinum toxin into the posterior crico-arytenoid muscles. Even more uncommonly known is cricothyroid muscle dystonia. This we have seen once, documented with laryngeal EMG, in a patient who tightens up to the point of vocal spasm only when singing in upper ranges.

Currently, many patients with SD are obtaining relief with localized botulinum toxin injections into the vocal folds, which causes a temporary paresis and denervation of the vocal fold muscles. The exact mechanism by which this treatment disrupts the spasmodic activity is not yet understood, however, it has been demonstrated as effective with most patients for periods of from three to six months, at which time the treatment is usually repeated [2].

Benign essential tremor is often familial and usually begins in late middle age. The family history is positive in 50%. It is characterized by rhythmic contractions of alternating muscle groups producing a tremorous shake that may affect the voice, hands, or head. Some feel that the tremor tends to start in the dominant hand and then spread to the voice. Benign essential tremor may be relatively spasm free, or combine with an element of spasm that makes for confusion with other forms of spasmodic dysphonias, so we may refer to tremor with spasm, or without.

Unfortunately, persons with essential voice tremor do not receive the same dramatic relief from botulinum toxin injections as those with dystonic spasm even though the spasm component of mixed tremor–spasm can be helped. The tremor component is often relieved by β-blockers such as propranolol in doses that may be gradually increased by up to 40 mg four times daily.

Parkinson's disease or other degenerative neurological disorders involve typical changes in voice function but do not generally present primarily as a voice disorder. The drug and neurological management of Parkinson's disease is beyond the scope of this book, but it should be pointed out that voice therapy can be quite useful in increasing vocal power and projection, thus avoiding the typical parkinsonian voice.

It may be helpful to consider a list of voice profiles associated with dystonia and tremor as follows:

- Adductor spasmodic dysphonia
- Adductor spasm with tremor (spasm predominant)
- Essential tremor with spasm (tremor predominant)
- Benign essential tremor
- Abductor spasmodic dysphonia (posterior crico-aryteroid)
- Singer's spasmodic dysphonia (cricothyroid)
- Adductor breathing dystonia
- Dysphonia with other dystonias (e.g. Meige's syndrome).

Having progressed through the decision tree it is likely that the diagnosis will have become fairly clear, and a treatment plan can logically follow. But, as has been discussed in other chapters, a dysphonia often has multiple causes and therefore requires multiple therapies. For example, a viral infection may trigger a technical muscle misuse, but a predisposing factor may have been gastric reflux and a perpetuating factor may be psychological stress or conflict. All aspects of the etiology need to be addressed in the treatment plan.

References

1. Arnold, G.E. (1962), Vocal rehabilitation of paralytic dysphonia. *Archives of Otolaryngology*, **76**, 358–68.

2. Blitzer A., Brin M. F., Fahn S. and Lovelace R.E. (1988) Localized injections of botulinum toxin for the treatment of focal laryngeal dystonia (spastic dysphonia). *Laryngoscope*, **98**, 193–7.

3. Bouchayer M., Cornut G., Witzig E. *et al*. (1985) Epidermoid cysts, sulci, and mucosal bridges of the true vocal fold: a report of 157 cases. *Laryngoscope*, **95**, 1087–94.

4. Crumley R.L., Izdebski K. and McMicken B. (1988) Nerve transfer versus teflon injection for vocal fold paralysis: a comparison. *Laryngoscope*, **98**, 1200–3.

5. Ford C.N. and Bless D.M. (1986) Injectable collagen in vocal fold augmentation: a preliminary clinical study. *Otolaryngology Head and Neck Surgery*, **94**, 104–12.

6. Isshiki N., Okamura H. and Ishikawa T. (1975) Thyroplasty type 1 (lateral compression) for dysphonia due to vocal fold paralysis or atrophy. *Acta Otolaryngological*, **80**, 465–73.

7. Morrison M.D. & Morris B.D. (1990). Dysphonia and bulimia: vomiting laryngeal injury. *Journal of Voice*, **4**, 76–80.

8. Olson N.R. (1991) Laryngopharyngeal manifestations of gastroesophageal reflux disease. *Otolaryngologic Clinics of North America*, **24** (5), 1201–13.

4

Approaches to voice therapy

4.1 PURPOSE OF THERAPY

The purpose of a voice therapy program varies from patient to patient. In most cases, the intent is to improve vocal communication, and in some cases to normalize voice function, that is to restore function so that the vocal profile falls within an accepted normal range. When pathogenesis includes irreversible or degenerative organic pathology, voice therapy may be initiated to maintain the current level of function as long as possible and reduce ineffective compensatory behaviors. When surgery or other medical intervention is selected as the primary management approach, pre-operative voice therapy may be undertaken to eliminate vocal abuses and provide models for optimizing postoperative voice. Postoperative therapy programs are designed to facilitate patients' adaptation to structural changes, and to optimize results of medical–surgical procedures with technical fine-tuning. In an ideal world of health care, the primary purpose of voice therapy programs for occupational and professional voice users would be to prevent dysphonias related to voice abuse and misuse. An important component of the voice therapy program is diagnostic therapy, which ideally takes place during the interdisciplinary evaluation period, so is discussed in detail in Chapter 1.

4.2 FACTORS INFLUENCING SELECTION AND SUCCESS OF THERAPY PROGRAMS

Voice therapy programs may consist primarily of short-term symptomatic techniques, or may encompass long-term comprehensive rehabilitation strategies. The choice of approaches and duration of the program depends on clinical, personal and economic factors. In general, individuals experiencing muscle misuse or psychogenic voice disorders with gradual onset, long-term, and consistent symptoms require longer, more comprehensive treatment protocols than those whose onset was sudden, with short-term and intermittent symptoms. Patients who have experienced gradual dysphonia onset are more likely to demonstrate generalized muscle misuse, during speech and nonspeech activities. Further, considerable adaptation may take place during a gradual onset, so an individual comes to accept the sounds and sensations of his or her disordered voice production as 'normal'. At this point, a muscle misuse voice disorder is habituated, a patient's awareness of muscle tension is minimized, and so too is the ability to correct inappropriate behaviors. Presence of a primary or secondary organic component may complicate prognosis and influence the choice of therapy techniques. If a long-standing lesion is present in the larynx, for example, a fibrotic nodule, compensatory behaviors may have developed and been reinforced as part of an individual's day-to-day coping strategies. The same may hold true for organic tremor, laryngeal dystonia or other neurological or systemic diseases. In cases where medical or surgical intervention is indicated, pre-operative voice therapy may be introduced to reduce vocal abuses and inappropriate compensatory behaviors such as increased glottic resistance, splinting in the jaw and tongue and incoordinate breathing. Most patients with long-standing dysphonias benefit from a comprehensive voice rehabilitation program either as the primary treatment, or following medical/surgical intervention.

Other factors that influence therapy selection and prognosis include hearing impairment, other sensory deficits, external support, impact of the dysfunction on one's life and unresolved psychological conflicts or psychiatric disease.

4.3 SYMPTOMATIC THERAPY

The term **symptomatic therapy** implies that therapeutic techniques are selected to target a particular set of signs or symptoms of a voice disorder. An assumption may be made that correction of a primary sign or symptom leads the patient to more generalized, positive behavior changes, such as reduction of muscle tension during speech. For example, a principal sign of adolescent transitional voice disorder (ATVD) might include use of falsetto register, and a resultant speaking pitch that is too high for the age and gender of the individual. Psychogenic etiologies are often suspected in ATVD, and habituated misuse of laryngeal and paralaryngeal muscles is common. Symptomatic therapy might be introduced to facilitate use of a more appropriate pitch by eliciting and extending use of modal register phonation or a lower pitch target. In fact, often patients are better able to produce extreme patterns of phonation more readily than 'normal' patterns: when ATVD is related to chronic muscle misuse, glottic fry register may be easier to establish initially. The first stage of therapy may then focus on maximizing various acoustic and kinaesthetic aspects of the falsetto–glottic fry contrast. Initial successful behavior changes are then expanded and shaped into closer approximations of 'normal', in this case lower pitched modal register phonation. Since modal register is a more natural speaking mode, we expect that consistent use of the lower pitch results in more relaxed and efficient speech behaviors. Incidentally, should a primary psychogenic etiology be identified in a patient with ATVD, therapy may not be initiated until it is evident that underlying conflicts have resolved sufficiently so as not to stand in the way of patient motivation and compliance.

Symptomatic therapy, and all voice therapy for that matter, relies heavily on successful use of one or more feedback channels to assist in motor learning. These include the auditory, visual, and tactile–kinesthetic processing systems. Other prerequisites to successful therapy include adequate attention skills to process instructions and use feedback signals to change one's speech motor behaviors; and adequate memory for retrieval of information critical to effective practice and behavior changes.

Symptomatic therapy may take on several forms depending on the classification scheme and physiological theories held by the clinician, and biofeedback instruments available in the clinic. In the ATVD case outlined above, auditory feedback might be used primarily to effect pitch-production changes, using the clinician's voice or a musical instrument as a model. For a patient who is more successful with visual input, a dedicated device for visual feedback of f_0 might be used to reinforce approximations to a target pitch range. Using the same patient profile, a different clinician may note an elevated laryngeal posture during phonation, and choose a facilitation technique to adjust the posture as a symptomatic approach. Manual pressure on the larynx, or postural adjustments to the head and neck might be used initially to establish a lowered larynx position prior to and during phonation. Assuming the same patient has a clinical profile that includes long-standing muscle misuse (perhaps in association with chronic anxiety), a clinician might decide that a comprehensive long-term therapy program is more appropriate, in association with psychological intervention if necessary. An example of a comprehensive voice rehabilitation program is outlined in section 4.4. (A list of facilitation techniques used commonly for treating patients symptomatically is listed in Chapter 1, section 1.9.)

4.4 COMPREHENSIVE VOICE REHABILITATION PROGRAMS

Many of the voice patients seen in an interdisciplinary voice clinic are occupational voice users: teachers, business executives, attorneys, clergy, vocational instructors, waiters, customer representatives, and media personnel. These individuals have high voice demands, depend on their voices to conduct their jobs, often in difficult social/emotional and acoustic environments, yet rarely have training in vocal technique. Occupational voice users typically present with symptoms and signs of vocal abuse/overuse, muscle misuse, dysphonia and often primary or secondary anxiety or depression. As busy professionals, some individuals may rely heavily on caffeine, have poor dietary habits, conduct business in noisy environments, and on the run. These lifestyle features may contribute further to poor vocal health by adding dehydration, anxiety, reflux laryngitis, and vocal abuse to the etiological profile.

Clearly, successful vocal rehabilitation with occupational voice users needs to address all the lifestyle, emotional and technical issues that are represented in a complex system of symptom formation. The methods presented here also serve as a useful outline for preventative programs, the ultimate health care goal for this particularly susceptible population. Most individuals respond well to a group therapy format for comprehensive voice rehabilitation. The group therapy approach has the advantages of saving time and money for the health care system or the patient, or both, and providing a venue for problem solving, desensitizing, and carry-over of techniques through peer-monitoring and role-playing exercises.

Comprehensive voice management ideally involves interdisciplinary program coordination, including input from the speech-language pathologist, psychiatrist, singing teacher, otolaryngologist and physical therapist, or posture specialist. The minimal components of a comprehensive voice rehabilitation program are listed below.

4.4.1 Education

Education provides basic information on speech physiology, vocal health issues and responses of the system to psychological and physical stressors. Although education can be an ongoing process in the program, core information is presented early.

4.4.2 Problem Solving

Problem solving is practised to learn strategies for adjusting environmental conditions leading to vocal abuse and postural misuse; and to practice stress management, by incorporating relaxation, work delegation, etc. This is an ongoing component of the program. Initially topics are introduced by the clinician(s), but later issues are often raised by patients as they become more aware of external and internal factors contributing to optimal or inappropriate voice use.

4.4.3 Relaxation Training

Relaxation training includes programs such as Jacobson's Progressive Relaxation[12]; or other cognitive or image-based exercises. This is also an ongoing learning process, but ideally introduced as one of the earliest technical training activities.

4.4.4 Alignment–Posture Training

Alignment–Posture training includes basic principles of proper alignment for the whole body to reduce muscle misuses, and ensure freedom of the respiratory, phonatory, resonance, and articulatory systems. Common theoretical perspectives guiding the training program include the Alexander technique [3] and the Feldenkrais method [10]. A specially-trained instructor may be engaged to train patients in a particular method. A physical therapist specializing in problems of the back and neck can provide valuable information in the group therapy format, and may be used as a referral source for individuals experiencing specific chronic symptoms of postural misuse or disease. The figures in Appendix B demonstrate basic aspects of the Alexander technique used by the speech pathologist, singing teacher and psychiatrist in this interdisciplinary clinic. Since specific relaxation training and optimal voice use depends on balanced posture, this training is introduced early in the sequence of components.

It is virtually impossible to experience coordination between the respiratory and phonatory systems for voice onset activities if the abdomen is held tightly; similarly passive jaw mobility during phonation cannot be established if the head is chronically retracted on the neck. Therefore, balanced posture is a pre-requisite to more focused therapy activities.

4.4.5 Specific Relaxation Exercises

Specific relaxation exercises are introduced based on individual needs. Commonly, patients require training in relaxation of the abdomen, shoulders, neck, face, jaw, tongue, and pharynx. Tension-reduction strategies may incorporate visual and kinesthetic feedback and cognitive imaging. In addition, biofeedback devices may be useful in early training stages. Flexibility and independent movement of articulators during speech is an ultimate goal for many of the specific relaxation protocols. This ensures that articulatory postures and movements do not impose undue postural constraints on the larynx during phonation, nor minimize resonance potential. These exercises may be introduced prior to phonation exercises; however, they are continued throughout the program in association with exercises for voice onset and extension of phonation.

4.4.6 Co-ordinated Voice Onset

Co-ordinated voice onset exercises are introduced to maximize onset control and power while minimizing extraneous voice-onset gestures in the larynx, such as hyperadduction leading to glottal attacks, or hypoadduction leading to breathy onsets. Examples of traditional voice onset exercises for hyperadducting behaviors include use of simulated 'yawn–sigh'; or imagined insertion of the glottic fricative /h/ in word or phrase-initial positions. Most patients respond well to a technique that uses 'spontaneous' vocalizations: /hm/, as in the affirmative /m hm/, which can be elicited with a good clinical model in virtually everyone, and lends itself well to the current theories of speech-breathing control (Appendix B, section B.5). The majority of patients immediately acknowledge kinesthetic awareness of lower thoracic-abdominal muscle activity when they employ a coordinated voice onset. Flexible endoscopy has revealed a reduction in magnitude of posterior glottic chinks in patients with laryngeal muscle misuse while they are employing this technique. It may contribute to more efficient voice production in patients with muscular tension dysphonias, as demonstrated by this laryngoscopic sign, as well as reduced mean phonatory flow rates and breathy perceptions [23, 24].

The coordinated voice onset has also been used successfully to optimize voice onset strategies in individuals with spasmodic dysphonias, and for a variety of organic problems leading to incompetent glottic closure. Once the basic onset technique is established, it can be extended to train use of respiratory 'support' for sustained sounds, intensity dynamics, and then speech phrases.

4.4.7 Resonance Enhancement

Resonance enhancement exercises are introduced to improve vocal tone, clarity and power. Patients are trained to maximize vocal resonance, initially by attending to kinesthetic sensations associated with sympathetic vibration of the vocal tract resonators. Nasal phonemes are often used to introduce the kinesthetic learning because of the distinct sensations associated with resonance in the nasal cavities. This kinesthetic awareness is used as a reference for vowels and other non-nasal voiced phonemes. Relaxed articulatory movements of the jaw, tongue, and lips are incorporated to facilitate maximum oral resonance sensations in a variety of sound sequences, then during speech. Relationships are sought between perceived resonance power and activity of the respiratory muscles, which in a sense, 'feed' the vocal tract resonators, by ensuring continuous air flow through the glottis. Guidelines provided by Lessac [17] and Linklater [18] are used for optimizing vowel resonance.

4.4.8 Vocal Flexibility

Vocal flexibility exercises are introduced to establish techniques for rapid pitch and intensity changes without muscle misuse. This stage of training targets effective intonation and linguistic stress in speech, and basic dynamics of singing. Initially, general and specific relaxation exercises are combined with 'vocal eases' often used in singing pedagogy, such as glissandos during lip and tongue trills, and 'siren' imitations. Patients are encouraged to apply the techniques to pitch and intensity dynamics during speech, and may use information from the clinician, each other and/or instrumental feedback to confirm dynamic range increases.

4.4.9 Generalization

Generalization to speech or vocal performance, or both, is the ongoing process of applying new techniques to real-life situations. Ideally, patients incorporate new behaviors during day-to-day communication at each stage of rehabilitation, so the final stage of therapy can focus on trouble-shooting in difficult situations. For example, early in the program, techniques are trained for establishing balanced posture, and these are practised intensively until the optimal behaviors predominate in everyday activities, and become 'automatic'. Balanced posture then becomes a prerequisite for good speech and singing regardless of what other techniques are being learned or applied concurrently. In the group therapy format, peer review and role playing serve as useful practice activities for generalization. Ultimately, each individual needs a method to monitor his or her vocal 'performance' on an ongoing basis. The clinician may participate by means of on-site evaluation with or without review of video tapes of a patient communicating or performing in typical situations. Each patient is expected to use vocal 'warm-up' and 'cool-down' regimens daily. The warm-up activities may be selected on an individual basis from the repertoire of techniques employed successfully during the rehabilitation program. Vocal performers are encouraged to recommence or continue an appropriate vocal pedagogical program.

4.5 THERAPY FOR SPECIAL VOICE DISORDER POPULATIONS

4.5.1 Interdisciplinary Management for Patients with Organic Disorders: Optimizing Function

Many individuals with primary organic voice disorders may benefit from pre- and postoperative voice therapy. Since all patients consulting the voice-disorder clinic undergo a comprehensive voice evaluation as described in Chapter 1, it should be clear when voice therapy is indicated as an adjunct to medical/surgical treatment. As part of the general evaluation, diagnostic therapy is initiated to determine an individual's potential for change with voice therapy as the primary treatment. When the evaluation results in recommendation for medical/surgical intervention, the primary goals of pre-operative therapy include reduction of vocal abuses and muscular misuses identified during evaluation, and elimination of ineffective compensatory behaviors that have developed in the presence of organic disease. Postoperatively, therapy focuses on techniques that facilitate adaptation to medical/surgical changes, and that optimize the effectiveness of the primary treatment. A comprehensive voice rehabilitation program may be recommended for individuals suffering voice dysfunction due to neurogenic/organic diseases that are not successfully treated with medical/surgical management. Even in the presence of permanent vocal fold incompetence or asymmetry, or muscle weakness in respiratory, articulatory or resonance mechanisms, optimal use of the various systems involved in voice production can result in improved functional communication, such as in patients with Parkinson's disease [21, 22].

4.5.2 Role of Voice Therapy for Treatment of Spasmodic Dysphonias

Speech/voice therapy for patients experiencing spasmodic dysphonia (SD) may be undertaken as a primary or secondary treatment. Primary treatment programs are those that focus on behavioral management techniques as the first or dominant symptom-reduction strategy. Secondary speech therapy is used as an adjunct to other surgical, medical or psychological treatment programs to enhance the primary treatment.

Primary voice therapy is generally intensive and long term, lasting from six months to two years, with daily, bi-weekly or weekly sessions. As with all disorders, diagnostic therapy is undertaken initially to determine a patient's ability to alter SD symptoms under controlled conditions, and to specify technical approaches that may be useful in achieving symptom reduction, before a voice therapy program is recommended as the primary treatment approach. Since the pathogenesis of SD may include primary or secondary psychological components, an interdisciplinary management program is often advantageous, and psychiatric evaluation and treatment may be a prerequisite to successful voice therapy [1]. Primary voice therapy is most successful with patients who have minimal associated tremor, for whom psychological conflicts have been resolved, and in whom symptoms have recent onset and are incipient.

The long-term voice therapy program encompasses holistic or symptomatic protocols, or both, that reduce primary symptoms of laryngeal hypervalving, and secondary symptoms exacerbating communication attempts: respiratory overloading and incoordination, head retraction, facial tension and tics, jaw and tongue splinting, pitch lowering, avoidance and linguistic editing. Various types of biofeedback (EMG, videolaryngoscopy, EGG, aerodynamic monitoring) may be used to supplement motor learning. Many aspects of behavioral management may resemble those used for treating speech fluency disorders. In addition, the therapy program usually incorporates psychological support and counseling, sometimes in cooperation with a consulting psychologist or psychiatrist. Examples of holistic techniques used in voice therapy include:

- Alexander technique
- Progressive relaxation [12]
- Chewing approach [11]
- Yawn–sigh approach.

Symptomatic techniques used include:

- Coordinated voice onset/lower lung volumes
- Easy voice onset/breathy voice
- Forward or neutral tongue positioning
- Forward resonance focus/humming
- Inhalation phonation [26]
- Passive jaw movements
- Pitch register therapy [2]
- Sound prolongation

Selection of symptomatic techniques is guided by specific phonatory characteristics of an individual's dysphonia, especially the primary nature of laryngeal spasms: adductory or abductory.

Secondary voice therapy is an important adjunct to medical/surgical SD intervention techniques. The current most popular primary treatment for SD is botulinum toxin injection to the intrinsic laryngeal muscles thought to be most involved in spasmodic activity: generally the thyro-arytenoid for primary adductory spasms, and the PCA for primary abductory spasms. Resection of the recurrent laryngeal nerve (RLN) is still used as a treatment for so-called 'adductor' SD in some centres, and laser reduction of vocal fold tissue may be used as a secondary surgical treatment in cases of symptom recurrence following RLN resection. Both of these techniques result in an acute period of weak and breathy voice. Return of stronger voice is inevitable with botulinum toxin treatments since it creates only temporary symptom reduction, but some patients undergoing RLN resection have permanently weak voices.

Voice therapy techniques may be trained prior to medical/surgical intervention to help patients reduce secondary behavioral symptoms before treatment. Pre- or postoperative voice therapy, or both, using approaches such as those listed above may enhance and prolong the effects of primary medical/surgical treatments such as botulinum toxin injections, or may be used to facilitate transition through the acute breathy voice stage immediately post-treatment. For patients who have undergone

RLN resection and other secondary permanent procedures, adjunctive therapy may be undertaken to optimize communication in the presence of chronic postsurgical vocal weakness.

4.5.3 Voice Therapy for Gender Dysphoria

The challenge facing gender dysphoria (transsexual) patients and their voice management team is a complex one. Colton and Casper [8] have suggested that the most immediate problem relates to inappropriate pitch. Since the male larynx is larger, with the membranous vocal folds longer by a factor of 1.3–1.6 [13, 31], it is obvious that the natural fundamental frequencies of male and female structures will tend to disclose the pretransitional sex of an adult. As Colton and Casper point out, this problem is minimized in female-to-male transitions with administration of male hormones, since vocal fold mass is an expected result of this treatment. However, individuals undergoing male-to-female transitions represent the majority of patients consulting the voice clinic, and administration of female hormones has no demonstrated effect of raising f_0.

The fundamental rate of vocal fold vibration affecting pitch perception is only one of several factors differentiating male from female voices. The average adult male vocal tract is of course considerably larger than that of women, but the size differences are not linear. For example, in addition to having longer vocal tracts, males have proportionally larger pharyngeal cavities [15]. Both size and shape differences contribute to formant frequencies which undoubtedly affect a listener's perception of 'maleness' or 'femaleness'.

Perceptual studies of gender identification support the notion that glottic source and vocal tract filter functions contribute to these judgments. Coleman studied acoustic influences on sex identification by providing an electronic larynx as the vibratory source for speech, with male subjects employing fundamental frequency in the female range and female subjects using a male frequency [8]. Although female's voices were misidentified as male based on a male f_0 range, Coleman concluded that listeners must have employed vocal tract resonance characteristics to correctly identify the sex of most male subjects, since their mechanically produced f_0 was biased in the female direction. Of course, the absence of feminine voice quality features associated with the glottic source waveform may have influenced judgements as well. Subsequent studies of transsexuals have suggested that a complex relationship exists between speech f_0, vocal tract size, and voice quality in the determination of sex identity judgements [7, 29].

Recent studies have investigated voice-quality differences between men and women, which may affect sex identification judgments [6, 16, 19]. These differences are generated by both voice source and vocal tract filter mechanisms. Structural features and social conditioning may contribute to larger posterior glottic chinks and shorter closed phases during the phonatory cycle in many women. Voices of North American women are typically perceived as 'breathy' by professional listeners and visitors to the continent. This perceptual feature can be largely accounted for by postural and vibratory characteristics in the larynx [16, 23, 28]. The acoustic effects of phonation with variable glottic chinks and open-to-closed phase ratios also can be seen in the vocal tract filter function for women. Both f_0 and glottic posture may contribute to greater harmonic–formant interaction, and less distinct formant frequencies [7, 15].

Therapeutic strategies to feminize the speech of male-to-female transsexual patients must account for both glottic source and vocal tract adjustments. In addition, male–female differences in articulatory style, suprasegmental features, vocabulary and pragmatics must be considered to optimize results. Of course non-linguistic gestures may also facilitate feminine perceptions, and these seem often to develop vicariously.

Therapy activities for the transsexual patient include techniques to alter pitch and register use, unless pharmaceutical or phonosurgical approaches are planned as primary treatments to change pitch. Individuals using a speaking f_0 range at or above 160 Hz are identified more often as 'female', other factors being held constant [29]. Visual feedback devices are often useful to assist patients in establishing and maintaining a higher or lower fundamental frequency. Most patients learn the 'breathy' quality well by imitating the therapist or a desired model. A caveat to therapy introduced to alter glottic source characteristics such as f_0 and glottic closure/voice quality: it is not yet clear to what extent alterations in these characteristics comprise normal variations in use of the larynx during discourse or alternatively, contribute to misuse of muscles. The clinician should incorporate exercises to monitor and reduce potentially hazardous muscle tension throughout the program. This may require use of flexible or rigid laryngoscopy and video stroboscopy to identify the nature of glottic postures associated with acoustic changes, and subsequent effects on vibratory characteristics.

Some patients may be able to adopt an altered laryngeal posture during speech, for example, an elevated larynx to shorten the resonance tract and raise formant frequencies. This maneuver may also effectively narrow the pharyngeal cavity, which is known to be larger in men. Biofeedback may be useful to establish these changes. This may include tactile monitoring of larynx position, visual monitoring with a mirror, or use of more sophisticated visual feedback equipment such as spectrograms that provide information about formant frequencies. Vocal tract length and formant frequencies may be affected by facial postures: for example slight lip retraction may compliment an elevated larynx and further decrease vocal tract length. Any adjustments recommended should be small, and they should be pursued only if the therapist can incorporate hygienic muscle use so that discomfort and vocal misuse will not develop as a result of posturing changes.

Anecdotal reports have suggested that male-to-female transsexuals who have been living as women for some time tend to develop slightly forward articulatory postures. This style may be accompanied and complimented by slight elevation of the larynx.

The therapy program may include work on intonation and stress patterns, which may influence impressions of 'maleness' and 'femaleness', in particular the tendency for females to have wider ranges of intonation has been demonstrated [25, 30, 32].

Vocabulary changes may also provide cues to the intended gender. As with nonlinguistic gestures, this characteristic seems to be learned vicariously in most individuals as they adjust to their changing gender roles.

Individuals suffering gender dysphoria are faced with ongoing physical, psycho-social and economic stress. These factors greatly increase their susceptibility to reactive muscle misuse. The voice use profiles of many transsexuals may reflect this susceptibility, so specific relaxation exercises need to be incorporated at all stages of the voice rehabilitation program. The voice-care team needs to remain sensitive to the lifestyle dynamics of these patients in order to determine treatment priorities. A voice therapy program demands considerable time and motivation and, in some cases, a large financial commitment. It is therefore critical that this portion of an individual's rehabilitation be timed appropriately so that he or she is not further distressed by unsuccessful treatment.

4.5.4 Communication Rehabilitation following Laryngectomy

Individuals who undergo ablative surgery to the larynx require an interdisciplinary approach to rehabilitation. Ideally, the team approach is adopted prior to surgery, when a patient is still able to express emotions and request information with the speech mechanism intact. Psychological counseling is an ongoing aspect of rehabilitation, and often becomes part of the speech pathologist's role. Speech and voice rehabilitation may be expedited if the psychologist or psychiatrist can provide expertise to facilitate a patient's psychosocial adjustment postsurgically. Peer group support systems are also invaluable during the critical period of emotional healing.

It is the primary responsibility of the speech pathologist to ensure that each patient has an adequate means of communication to express practical and emotional needs during the adjustment period. Ultimately, the speech pathologist endeavours to provide each individual with information and training in the most effective method for communication.

Patients must of course make their own choices regarding voice restoration techniques that require further surgical intervention, such as tracheo-esophageal puncture (TEP). Before such a procedure is selected as a primary management strategy, the speech pathologist and otolaryngologist together present surgical options, prognosis, and risk factors determined by individual patient profiles. Patients who are offered secondary TEP intervention approach are pre-selected based on criteria adapted from Blom and Singer [4, 27].

- Patient expresses motivation to improve communication.
- Patient demonstrates adequate self-care skills to maintain stoma/TEP hygiene: eyesight; manual/digital dexterity.
- Patient demonstrates realistic expectations regarding speech outcome.
- Tracheostoma is not situated inferior to sternal notch.
- Patient can phonate fluently during transnasal insufflation test: 8 s /a/; count to 10.
- Stoma is not less than 2 cm at its widest point.
- No medical contraindications to surgery or TEP method exist.

In instances where TEP or other surgical voice restoration procedures are not medically or surgically viable, or where eligible patients elect not to undergo this procedure, other options for effective communication are explored. These include esophageal voice training, use of electronic or pneumatic speech aids, and other augmentative communication systems.

Whenever possible, family and friends are included in the communication rehabilitation program. This allows the team to provide support and education for the patient and family together. Communication partners are trained to adapt to an alternative set of speech/voice/communication systems, and to be effective 'listeners' and communication facilitators. For more comprehensive information on techniques of communication rehabilitation of patients following ablative surgery, the reader is referred to current texts on this topic [5, 9, 14, 20].

4.5.5 Voice Therapy for Children: Special Considerations:

Voice management for the pediatric population demands special consideration of the role that care-givers, educators, and peers play in influencing a child's behavior. Aspects of development, evaluation and etiology of voice disorders in children are presented in detail in a separate chapter (Chapter 7).

In the child with a severe congenital disorder impairing voice function, the speech language pathologist may provide counseling to parents and other care-givers regarding the best ways to ensure that the child has access to sensory experiences thought to be prerequisite to cognitive and linguistic development. If nonvocal communication is to be longterm, then all appropriate augmentative and alternative methods should be explored to provide the most effective and efficient expression of the child's needs and thoughts.

Voice therapy to remediate abusive vocal behaviors or muscle misuse voice disorders should involve cooperation of family, educators, peer, and friends as appropriate. In instances where vocally aggressive behavior (or conversely, reduced vocal dynamics) is an expression of a need for the child to gain control over his social or home environment, the origin of the psychosocial needs should be explored. In some cases, the community or school psychologist or psychiatrist may be included in evaluation and counseling of the child and family when a difficult psychosocial dynamic exists.

Direct therapy with children may be appropriate in cases where the family, educators, and other significant persons can attend treatment sessions to provide support and carry-over. In general, for children under the age of eight or nine years, or for the immature, dependent child, a home-based or school-based program, or both, that integrates new vocal behaviors into the child's everyday activities will be most successful. In such cases, the family, with or without the teacher, is trained to adopt the primary role as therapist. As such the care-giver provides appropriate models for voice production; helps the child monitor his or her own behavior; participates in vocal games and exercises to reinforce good posture and vocal use; and supports the child's attempts to modify behavior. When behavior changes are required during activities with peers, such as sporting events or group discussions, the entire 'team' may be educated and involved in appropriate voice use. In this situation, the important peer influence may become a supportive and integrated one, rather than a factor precipitating or perpetuating abusive vocal behavior. Further, peer involvement in an indirect voice therapy program relieves the stigma for the voice-disordered child, and may provide vicarious learning of more effective communication skills for all participants.

The long-term efficacy of therapy for children with mild dysphonia related to vocal nodules is unfortunately not well documented. Although anecdotal reports suggest that nodules regress spontaneously in boys after puberty, the muscle misuses that often accompany and may be the primary cause of these lesions can persist into adulthood if not treated. Further, in some cases, the presence of a mild dysphonia may represent a variety of organic or psychosocial problems, or both, which require attention so as not to negatively affect communication development in the long term.

4.5.6 Principles and Voice Techniques for Treating Patients with Conversion Dysphonia/Aphonia

The primary approach in voice therapy for individuals suffering conversion dysphonias/aphonias may be symptomatic, particularly if symptoms are recent, and precipitating psychological conflicts have resolved. The program is generally short term. In most cases, full restoration of voice is the goal for the first therapy session, followed by brief follow-up visits or telephone conversations.

If therapy is undertaken on the same day as the evaluation, supportive family members or friends who may have accompanied the patient to the clinic are encouraged to attend the therapy session. If therapy is scheduled for a subsequent day, the patient is requested to bring a supportive friend or family member.

Typical goals and activities

Education and sound introduction

The patient is reassured by the consulting physician and speech pathologist that no structural abnormalities or disease processes are present to account for the dysphonia. Most patients seek reassurance that no carcinoma or other life-threatening diseases are present. If an upper respiratory tract infection coincided with dysphonia onset, the patient must often be convinced that no residual signs are present to threaten voice recovery. Samples of the videolaryngostroboscopic exam are reviewed with the patient to reinforce the clinicians' reports and to demonstrate evidence of 'normal' voice function, for example during cough, sigh, or inhalation phonation.

The clinician describes relevant principles of normal phonation, and the specific mechanisms of muscle misuse that result in the patient's dysphonia. The final common pathway: muscle misuse, is emphasized as the mechanism of dysfunction, not psychopathology.

The clinician describes and demonstrates mechanical adjustments that are necessary to produce normal phonation. If diagnostic therapy has not yet been undertaken to determine which techniques facilitate change most effectively, it is incorporated at this stage. The nature of the techniques selected, and explanation for their success depends on observations made during the diagnostic therapy probes. For a comprehensive list of techniques see section 1.9 in Chapter 1.

Examples of explanations to effect change include:

- *Problem*: vocal folds hyperabducted (held open tightly).
  Solution: adduct (close) the vocal folds to phonate.
  How?: cough; throat-clear; hum; push/pull; squeak at high pitch; use low-pitched glottic fry phonation; inhalation phonation; sigh; laugh; manipulate larynx . . .
- *Problem*: vocal folds and/or ventricular folds hyperadducted.
  Solution: relax the vocal tract and vocal folds.
  How?: yawn; sigh; breathy voice; inhalation phonation; alter target pitch; phonation with simultaneous head, shoulder, jaw movements; manipulate larynx . . .
- *Problem*: vocal folds inconsistently adducted.
  Solution: feel the sound consistently.
  How?: palpate larynx during phonation to gain kinesthetic awareness of resonance . . .

When generalized muscle and postural misuse is present during phonation attempts, holistic and specific relaxation exercises may be introduced to increase success with voice restoration. Sample exercises are outlined in Appendix B.

Once a facilitation exercise has been applied successfully to initiate phonation, the patient is encouraged to combine this technique with sound extension, typically a vowel or nasal phoneme /m/. Tactile, auditory and visual feedback devices may be used to provide information regarding phonation consistency. At this point, the clinician and support person provide reinforcement and encouragement generously. The first attempts at extending phonation may not represent the patient's normal phonation style, but he or she is reassured that a more natural style will develop, and tactics are introduced to shape the sound production.

Guidelines for shaping sound extension
If the patient's dysphonic voice sounds too high-pitched and squeaky, a glissando pitch change with continuous phonation may facilitate transition to a lower pitch. Alternatively, glottic fry register might be employed to experience lower-pitched phonation, with maximum kinesthetic feedback from the larynx. When pitch or intensity of consistent glottic fry phonation are increased, a transition into modal register generally occurs.

If the patient's voice sounds too low-pitched, phonation in falsetto register might be introduced to interrupt the misuse pattern. High pitched phonation on /i/ (*ee*) or /u/ (*oo*) may be most successful. A siren imitation may ease the transition to a more appropriate pitch range (Appendix B, Section B.7.2). Also, exercises designed to increase oral resonance often facilitate a more natural pitch range. Spontaneous vocalizations such as /hm/; /m hm/ may provide a pitch reference that is more appropriate (Appendix B, section B.5).

If the larynx tends to rise with phonation attempts, manual pressure or altered head position may be used to maintain an appropriate larynx posture.

Tactile kinesthetic feedback is useful to help the patient gain control over phonation consistency. Light palpation on the thyroid lamina region and on the nasal bone may provide the tactile feedback necessary for continuous phonation.

Once continuous relaxed phonation is achieved on a single sound in an appropriate pitch range, the clinician advises the patient that successful phonation techniques can be extended to all sound productions. Principles of articulation are discussed and simple relaxed tongue, jaw, lip and velar movements are introduced to practice sound transitions during sustained phonation, for example extending a hum-to-vowel transition: /mamamamamama/; /mimimimimimi/; /memememememe/; /momomomo-momo/; /mumumumumumu/; Some patients will recognize the speech approximation and spontaneously apply phonation to conversational use at this point. Others may require further coaching, and gradual approximations to recognizable speech. Transitional stages include multiple sound transitions on sustained phonation: /mamamimimama/; /nananunano/; /malamalama/; /namolunabe/. Voiceless pho-nemes may be introduced at a later stage, once consistent phonation is achieved on all-voiced sequences: /mapadapala/; /nesilamuta/. A few words and speech phrases may sneak into the sound sequences: /senotumi/. At this stage, distraction from the mechanics may be useful to allow for generalization of the phonation to speech. The support person may begin to recognize the speech phrases and react accordingly. Encouragement and praise are again generously offered to the patient who is required to continue with phonation exercises until he or she is confident enough to apply it to spontaneous speech. Serial speech may be introduced as a further transitional stage. (counting, reciting days of week, months of year, etc.) Responsibility to select and apply techniques is gradually transferred to the patient.

The patient, clinician and support person engage in conversation to build the patient's confidence, and to troubleshoot for potential problems. If inconsistency is noted, the patient is requested to select and apply a technique to facilitate a more appropriate phonation pattern, and coached as required. Suggestions are made for ongoing practice, generally at the nonsense syllable or serial speech stage, to build confidence and reinforce appropriate motor patterns. The patient and support person are instructed to continue conversing at home throughout the day. The patient is reassured that the restored voice represents the most natural and efficient method of speaking, and for that reason will be easy to maintain. Further information is exchanged with the patient and support person at their request.

A re-check phone conversation or office visit is scheduled for the following day, depending on the level of success achieved during the initial session. During follow-up phone calls, further office visits are scheduled as indicated by the patient's report and clinician's observations. The patient is encouraged to call immediately if any questions or concerns arise.

Prognostic Factors in Treatment of Psychogenic Dysphonias

The following questions need to be considered to establish treatment priorities and predict therapy outcome.

- Has the precipitating stressor/conflict been resolved? (Yes = positive prognosis).
- How long has the dysphonia persisted? (long duration = negative prognosis). How consistent are the symptoms? (consistent may, or may not = negative prognosis).
- Has the patient experienced unsuccessful treatment consultations prior to this one? (Yes = negative prognosis).
- Was the patient prescribed voice rest for the current problem? (Yes = negative prognosis).
- Is the patient self-assured that persistent somatic symptoms (muscle pain, globus pharyngeus, dysphonia) do not represent a serious and life-threatening medical problem such as cancer? (Yes = positive prognosis).
- Is the patient receiving attention or reinforcement as a result of the dysphonia (secondary gain)? (Yes = negative prognosis).
- Does the patient have confidence that you can help restore his or her voice today? (Yes = positive prognosis).

Indications for Psychiatric Referral

During a voice evaluation or treatment program, several factors may indicate that psychiatric consultation/intervention is necessary to improve prognosis for voice therapy. These are outlined below:

During initial evaluation:

- evidence in patient's history of psychiatric disorder;
- predisposing personality factors: narcissistic preoccupation with voice and/or perfect performance; inhibition of expression of assertiveness; inability to permit vocal crying; hypochondriacal traits; tendency to somatize psychological conflicts;
- coincidence of psychological stressors or 'event' and onset of dysphonia, where conflict is not clearly resolved;
- psychological distress concomitant with physical illness that commonly affects the voice (eg.'flu);
- patient consistently experiences anticipatory anxiety about voice production;
- cause and effect relationships unclear (Figure 4.1)
- patient requests psychiatric referral.

During voice therapy program:

- reduced patient motivation;
- inappropriate patient response to demonstrated voice improvement;
- recurrence of dysphonia following initial recovery;
- persistent signs of anxiety, depression, or psychological conflict;
- patient requests a psychiatry referral.

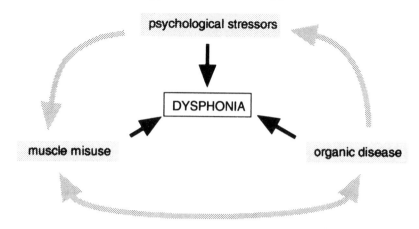

Figure 4.1 Interacting etiological factors in dysphonia symptom formation.

The reader is referred to Appendix B which includes protocol samples for training aspects of vocal hygiene; relaxation; posture alignment; specific relaxation; coordinated voice onset; resonance development and vocal flexibility. The protocols are presented in the format of patient practice worksheets, similar to those distributed to our patients to supplement the comprehensive voice rehabilitation program.

References

1. Aronson, A.E. (1985) *Clinical Voice Disorders An Interdisciplinary Approach*, 2nd Ed. Thieme, New York, NY.
2. Barkmeier, J. and Verdolini-Marston, K. (1992) Behavioral treatment for adductory spasmodic dysphonia. Handout distributed at the Second Biennial Phonosurgery Symposium, July, 1992, Madison, WI.
3. Barlow W. (1973) *The Alexander Technique*, Warner Books, New York, NY.
4. Blom E.D. and Singer M.I. (1979) Surgical-prosthetic approaches for postlaryngectomy voice rehabilitation, in *Laryngectomee Rehabilitation* (eds R.L. Keith and F.C. Darley), College-Hill, Houston, TK.
5. Casper J.K. and Colton (1992) *Clinical Manual for Laryngectomy and Head and Neck Cancer Rehabilitation*, Singular, San Diego, CA.
6. Coleman R.O. (1976) A comparison of the contributions of two voice quality characteristics to the perception of maleness and femaleness in the voice. *Journal of Speech and Hearing Research*, **19** 168–80.
7. Coleman R.O. (1971) Male and female voice quality and its relationship to vowel formant frequencies. *Journal of Speech and Hearing Research*, **14** 565–77.
8. Colton R.H. and Casper J.K. (1990) *Understanding Voice Problems. A Physiological Perspective for Diagnosis and Treatment*, Williams & Wilkins, Baltimore, MD.
9. Edels Y. (1983) *Laryngectomy: Diagnosis to Rehabilitation*, Aspens Systems, Rockville, MD.
10. Feldenkrais M. (1949) *Body and Mature Behaviour*, International University, New York, NY.
11. Froeschels E. (1952) Chewing method as therapy. *Archives of Otolaryngology*, **LVI** 427–34.
12. Jacobson E. (1938) *Progressive Relaxation*, 2nd edn, University of Chicago, Chicago, IL.

13. Kahane J.C. (1983) Postnatal development and aging of the human larynx. *Seminars in Speech and Language,* **4** (3) 189–203.

14. Keith R.L. and Darley F.L. (1979) *Laryngectomee Rehabilitation,* College-Hill, Houston, TX.

15. Kent R.D. and Read C (1992) *The Acoustic Analysis of Speech,* Singular, San Diego, CA.

16. Klatt D.H. and Klatt L.C. (1990) Analysis, synthesis and perception of voice quality variations among female and male talkers. *Journal of the Acoustic Society of America.* **87** (2) 820–57.

17. Lessac A. (1973) *The Use and Training of the Human Voice.* Drama, New York, NY.

18. Linklater K. (1976) *Freeing the Natural Voice,* Drama, New York, NY.

19. Nittrouer S., McGowan R.S., Milenkovic P.H., Beehler D. (1990) Acoustic measurements of men's and women's voices: a study of context effects and covariation. *Journal of Speech and Hearing Research,* **33** 761–75.

20. Prater R.J. and Swift R.W. (1984) *Manual of Voice Therapy,* Little Brown, Boston, MA.

21. Ramig L.O., Horii Y. and Bonitati C. (1991) The efficacy of voice therapy for patients with Parkinson's disease. *National Centre for Voice and Speech Status Progress Report,* National Centre for Voice and Speech, University of IOWA, IOWA City, ID, pp. 61–86.

22. Ramig L.O. and Scherer R.C. (1992) Speech therapy for neurologic disorders of the larynx, in *Neurologic Disorders of the Larynx* (eds. A. Blitzer, M. Brin, C. Susaki *et al.*) New York, NY, pp. 163–81.

23. Rammage L.A. (1992) Acoustic, aerodynamic and vibratory characteristics of phonation with variable posterior glottis postures. Doctoral dissertation, University of Wisconsin-Madison.

24. Rammage L.A., Morrison M.D. and Nichol H. (1986) *Muscular Tension Dysphonia* (videotape). Voice Foundation, New York, NY.

25. Richards D.M. (1975) A comparative study of the intonation characteristics of young adult males and females. Doctoral dissertation, Case Western Reserve University.

26. Shulman S. (1989) *Spasmodic Dysphonia: Techniques and Approaches in Successful Voice Therapy* American Speech – Language – Hearing Association, Rockville, MD.

27. Singer M.I. and Blom, E.D. (1980) An endoscopic technique for restoration of voice after laryngectomy. *Annals of Otology, Rhinology and Laryngology,* **89**, 529.

28. Sodersten M and Lindestad P-A (1990) Glottal closure and perceived breathiness during phonation in normally speaking subjects. *Journal of Speech and Hearing Research,* **33**(3), 601–11.

29. Spencer L.E. (1988) Speech characteristics of male-to-female transsexuals: a perceptual and acoustic study. *Folia Phoniatrica,* **40**, 31–42.

30. Terango L. (1966) Pitch and duration characteristics of the oral reading of males on a masculinity-femininity dimension. *Journal of Speech and Hearing Research,* **9** 590–5.

31. Titze I.R. (1989) Physiologic and acoustic differences between male and female voices. *Journal of the Acoustic Society of America,* **85**, 1699–707.

32. Wolfe V.I., Ratusnik D.L., Smith F.H. and Northrup G. (1990) Intonation and fundamental frequency in male-to-female transsexuals. *Journal of Speech and Hearing Disorders,* **55**, 43–50.

Further Reading

Andrews M.L. (1991) *Voice Therapy for Children,* Singular, San Diego, CA.

Moncur J.P. and Brackett I.P. (1974) *Modifying Vocal Behavior,* Harper & Row, New York, NY.

Wilson D.K. (1979) *Voice Problems of Children,* 2nd ed, Williams & Wilkins, Baltimore, MD.

5

Psychological management of the voice disordered patient

5.1 INTRODUCTION

The function of voice is principally to communicate with other people. It is thus seen to have a major social component that serves to disperse feelings of psychological isolation. In order to speak, one requires an organic apparatus capable of producing sound, a psychological intent to communicate, and a social context in which one feels the desire to talk, since most people do not talk much to themselves, they think instead. Voice production, therefore, clearly rests upon the outcome of the interaction of factors that can be conceptualized as being at organic, psychological, and social levels. These assertions are obvious and hardly warrant mention. What does require emphasis is the principle underlying all our work in the voice clinic. Namely, that human beings are constituted so that their functioning is the outcome of the constant interplay of thoughts, emotions and actions, the last being mediated by the voluntary musculature.

An individual's voice is a very sensitive indicator of emotions, attitudes, and role assumptions. It is therefore not surprising that impairments of voice function are not uncommon accompaniments of psychological conflicts. However, the factors producing a dysphonic voice are a complex mixture of organic and psychological features occurring in a social context. A relatively minor organic change such as edema, infection, polypoidal change, or neoplasia may trigger a functional misuse, in which most of the voice problem is of psychological origin. This is particularly likely to happen if there is another organic predisposing condition, such as reflux esophagitis and acid laryngitis. Similarly, psychologically and socially induced vocal and misuse may lead to a secondary laryngeal organic problem such polypoidal degeneration. For example, the hoarseness associated with an early cancer of the vocal fold may be due as much to the ventricular band dysphonia as to the malignancy itself. Interestingly, when the carcinoma is resolved after radiation, the dysphonia of psychological origin that was causing most of the hoarseness may also be improved; however, this dysphonia may persist and lead to continuing concern about the tumor still being present. In cases such as this it is easy to see that the assessment and management of patients with voice disorders has confronted clinicians with their limitations. Both the absence of more objective and standardized assessment tools and procedures, and the failure of professionals to use uniform diagnostic terminology have complicated our understanding of the problem.

5.2 BRIEF REVIEW OF THE LITERATURE

To go back in time no farther than Shakespeare who has Hamlet assert: 'Tears in his eyes, distraction in 's aspect, a broken voice. . .', we see recognition of a connection between emotionally laden ideas and a voice disorder. For more than a century aphonia and dysphonia have been associated with the psychiatric disorder of hysteria [17].

Although voice disorders are commonly seen in general medical practice [19], there are no epidemiological data on their incidence and prevalence. Dysphonias afflict individuals of all ages, women more often than men [6, 14]. Although no predominant predisposing personality types have been found to be linked to the symptom of dysphonia, earlier literature tended to emphasize the association with hysterical personality [3] while more recently a number of patients have been described as being introverted [11].

There is wide spread belief in the close association between personality traits and voice characteristics. Experimental confirmation was found that the voice did convey correct information concerning outer and inner characteristics of personality [2]. The same study showed, however, that there was not uniformity in the expression of personality through voice; rather, many features of many personalities can be determined from voice. The personality trait of dominance and the voice characteristics of loudness, resonance and lower pitch were found to be associated; submission, by contrast, was not [22]. This study supported the hypothesis that certain personality traits and certain voice characteristics may have developed together as reactions to situations involving social communication. One thinks of the modeling that parents provide for their children, not only vocal but also emotional and postural. The association of personal characteristics and emotion with the nonverbal properties of speech, including pitch, loudness and tempo, has been demonstrated [7, 15, 21, 23, 24]. The complexity of the effect of emotion on voice is readily to be recognized when one accepts that the human voice simultaneously conveys semantic content, momentary emotional states and the more enduring characteristics of the speaker, all modified by the social context in which the communication is taking place [10].

Theories of emotion abound but this publication is not the place for a detailed review of them. It is worth noting, however, that in a major publication on human emotions [18] there is no mention of the voice as a transmitter of emotion, whereas a substantial emphasis is given to facial expression as the supreme center of sending and receiving social signals. Each emotion is deemed to have an inherently adaptive function based upon a specific and innately determined neural substrate, a characteristic facial expression or neuromuscular expressive pattern, and a distinct subjective quality. What is true for the face as an organ of emotional expression is also true for the voice. Just as an individual's attitudes are entrenched in characteristic facial expressions and generalized body posture, as Alexander long ago made clear [1, 4, 5, 12], so will the muscles of phonation be programmed either to express emotions or to suppress them if doing so would be too anxiety provoking. This last point introduces the usefulness of the concept of state dependent memory, learning and behavior; significant psychological events impinging upon an individual, which arouse emotions and an impulse to action that are inhibited by anxiety, can serve to produce a state in which the muscle misuse becomes entrenched and can later be reactivated by the individual perceiving any feature of the earlier event, often outside the patient's full awareness [29, 30]. To seek to avoid awareness of such anxiety-provoking stimuli, whether from the environment or from within, patients heighten the recognition threshold thereby defending themselves from the perception which is then kept out of conscious awareness [8]. We see what it is safe to see and feel what we can permit ourselves to feel without distress.

This suppression of awareness of cues from the environment and proprioceptor sensations from within has the consequence of making individuals more emotionally wooden, and some of them dysphonic; this inability to respond emotionally has been termed **alexithymia** and has been associated with patients with psychosomatic disorder [20, 33].

Dysphonia may, and very often does, present in individuals who are free of clinical psychiatric disorder [13]. A study confirming our own findings of this in the voice clinic showed that two thirds of patients evaluated for functional dysphonia did not receive a psychiatric diagnosis [14]. Where psychiatric disorders are recognized they include major depression and dysthymic disorders, adjustment disorders with depression or anxiety, generalized anxiety disorder, conversion and phobic disorders, post-traumatic stress disorder, as well as personality trait difficulties. Only very occasionally was the dysphonia due to a schizophrenic disorder.

5.3 INDICATIONS FOR REFERRAL FOR PSYCHIATRIC CONSULTATION

The recognition by the otolaryngologist that the patient has a psychiatric disorder should prompt referral where the patient is not already seeing a psychiatrist. In a number of incidences evidence of formal psychiatric disorder is not forthcoming. Rather, personality factors that may predispose the patient to dysphonia are in evidence. These vary considerably and include a narcissistic preoccupation with voice, preoccupation with perfect performance, and a tendency to somatize psychological conflicts [31]. In addition, a number of patients show a marked inhibition in the expression of emotions; assertiveness, let alone the overt expression of anger, may be restrained, whereas other patients reveal an inability to permit themselves to cry. A hypochondriacal trait should not go unrecognized.

In taking the history from the patient it is important to note any psychological stressors which were impinging on the individual at the time of the onset of the disorder. This is particularly relevant where the psychological distress in the patient occurred concomitantly with the physical illness affecting the voice. Once a dysphonia has been present for a while, a carefully taken history will often reveal that the patient

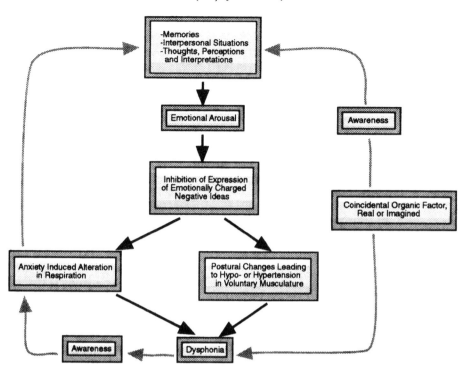

Figure 5.1 Mechanisms in the production of dysphonia.

experiences anticipatory anxiety about voice production, typified in such statements as: 'When the phone rings I just know my voice will not let me answer it.' In each of these cases the patient's attitude can lead to perpetuation of the dysphonia, which may require assistance of a psychiatrist for its resolution (Figure 5.1).

The approach to the evaluation and treatment of the voice disordered patient advocated in this text clearly requires the close collaboration of the otolaryngologist, speech pathologist, and psychiatrist. The context in which we work has made this possible for our patients; in Canada, universal medicare has eliminated all financial barriers to their access to treatment. Impediments remain, however, to the implementation of a satisfactory treatment plan. Speech pathologists and psychiatrists familiar with the management of voice disorders are in short supply and their distribution is such that many patients from smaller communities do not have ready access to them. Another factor often encountered is the attitude of a number of patients; having been relieved of the anxiety that they had cancer, a substantial proportion of them showed little motivation to carry out the exercises given by the speech pathologist or to clarify and resolve the psychological factors sustaining their dysphonia.

5.4 TYPES OF PATHOGENESIS OBSERVED IN DYSPHONIA OF
PSYCHOLOGICAL ORIGIN

Tensional symptoms arise from overactivity of the autonomic and voluntary nervous
systems in individuals who are unduly aroused and anxious. This leads to voluntary
muscle misuse, usually with generalized muscular hypertonicity. Specifically, hypertonicity of the intrinsic and extrinsic muscles of the larynx cause muscular tension
dysphonias; these are at times associated with psychiatric disorders such as adjustment
disorders and anxiety disorders, or with personality trait disturbances.

Symbolic symptoms occur on the basis of an unconscious substitution of a somatic
symptom involving the sensory or voluntary motor nervous system for a
psychological conflict. This is the conversion disorder referred to so frequently in the
psychiatric literature and gives rise to aphonia or dysphonia when the muscles involved
are those of phonation. Some recent work suggests the involvement of conscious
mechanisms in the production of conversion symptoms [16]. This should come as no
surprise to those working with dysphonic patients who have frequently seen a
substantial improvement in voice when the patient is distracted only to have a
deterioration occur when the patient again focused back on their voice difficulties.

Hypochondriacal symptoms, or the self-fulfilling anticipation of poor voice
production, occur in those who are unduly aware of, or responsive to, sensations arising
from a particular portion of their anatomy – in the case of those with dysphonias,
usually their mouth, throat and respiratory system. The associated psychiatric
diagnoses are often personality trait disturbances involving obsessive–compulsive and
dependent features, as well as hypochondriacal ones.

Depressive equivalent symptoms may arise in those individuals who are not
complaining overtly of depressive symptomatology but are suppressing the impulse to
cry or to express anger verbally. Adjustment, dysthymic and affective disorders of the
depressive type are the psychiatric diagnoses found in these cases.

A single patient may show symptoms of several categories such as those of
symbolic, tensional or hypochondriacal origin, at any particular time [25]. One type of
pathogenesis may reinforce another; for example, there may be a hypochondriacal
exaggeration of a tensional symptom. It is relevant to note these differing types of
pathogenesis since the treatment of the symptoms may well need to be different. And,
finally, organic and psychogenic processes are frequently combined and obviously
require differing therapeutic approaches [32].

The factors producing a dysphonic voice are often a complex mixture of organic,
psychological and social features, any one of which may be predisposing, precipitating
or perpetuating agents. Several case examples of this are provided at various points in
this text.

5.5 FUNCTION OF PSYCHOGENIC DYSPHONIA

The function of the symptom of psychogenic dysphonia may vary substantially from
patient to patient and these differences must be understood for therapy to be directed

appropriately. The term **primary gain** refers to the reduction of anxiety, tension and conflict which is provided by the production of a symptom of psychogenic origin, such as a dysphonia, through the employment of various defense mechanisms such as regression, repression, denial, reaction formation, and isolation of affect. Psychogenic dysphonia, although unpleasant in itself, constitutes for the patient a lesser evil than the personal problems from which it arose.

Case 1

A middle-aged woman had a respiratory tract infection which produced dysphonia while she was awaiting her triple-bypass cardiac surgery, about which she was very apprehensive. The infection resolved but her dysphonia persisted even after her operation, which she did not accept as having been as successful as her cardiologist asserted. Her husband kept saying to her: 'It is better to have a hoarse voice to worry about, rather than a bad heart', thereby helping to perpetuate the symptoms. At the clinic she was seen jointly by the otolaryngologist, the speech pathologist and the psychiatrist. In the presence of all three the otolaryngologist showed and discussed with her the videotape of her normal larynx. A sample of her voice was audiotaped, after which she was interviewed by the psychiatrist, during which her doubts about her heart operation as well as her reluctance to stand up to her domineering husband was recognized. 'As I get older it bothers me more that he is the decision maker. I'd like to have my voice back but it would only lead to more arguments.' She was encouraged to retrieve her voice and to take the risk. The psychiatrist met with the speech pathologist to pass on his findings before speech therapy was started. The husband was advised to change his behavior.

Secondary gain is the benefit derived by the individual from the external environment on the basis of the perception by others of his or her evident distress; this may take the form of monetary compensation, increased attention or sympathy, and the satisfaction of dependency needs. These secondary gains may serve to reinforce the patient's disorder and perpetuate its persistence.

Sociologists have emphasized that the assumption by an individual of the 'sick role' and the display of 'invalid behavior' may convey many valuable privileges. Invalids may not only be exempted from normal social obligations but they may also be freed from accounting for their responsibilities. Society requires the individual to seek appropriate treatment for his or her disability so that he or she exercises the privileges of the sick role for as brief a time as possible. Failure to do this is perceived correctly as the employment of the symptom for secondary gain.

Case 2

A school teacher with an obsessively perfectionist personality trait, coupled with a paranoid attitude, who was having difficulties in his marriage was confronted by an extremely defiant group of young adolescents whom he described as 'that class of destroyers trying to get me'. He would lose his voice for 5–15 minutes when he raised it to try to restore order in the classroom; his failure to succeed in doing so increased feelings of depression. Prior to attending the clinic he had been placed on long-term disability leave which would carry him through on full pay to retirement age. He was reluctant to accept speech therapy, to take medication or to engage in psychotherapy.

In appraising our patients and their response to treatment it is necessary to differentiate the extent to which the symptom of dysphonia has primary or secondary gain attributes, since this will influence the manner in which treatment needs to be directed. It is often necessary to alter the behavior of those in the patient's immediate social network in order to diminish the rewards conferred by the assumption of the sick role; this is frequently not easy to do.

Case 3

A 14-year-old high-school student was referred to the clinic because of episodes of aphonia which had led to his refusal to go to school; his mother had accepted this behavior. It emerged that he was his mother's only child and had never known his father. He had been brought up in the house of his maternal grandparents with his grandmother being his principal care-giver; she had been extremely indulgent of his every wish so that the description of him as a spoiled child was very accurate indeed. When his mother moved several hundred miles away with her son to be the housekeeper for a relative, the indulgent atmosphere to which he had been accustomed was lost in a household where other children also received consideration. On examination, it became evident that the boy was deliberately producing the dysphonia. At times he would refuse to respond at all, merely glaring at the otolaryngologist, the speech pathologist, or the psychiatrist. Nothing in the history obtained from the mother or in the examination of the boy, suggested the presence of a formal psychiatric disorder. He made it clear that his voice would undoubtedly return the moment he went back to live with his grandmother which his mother adamantly opposed. The grandparents were convinced that the boy was physically ill and would not drive him and his mother several miles to the clinic for his speech therapy and psychiatric follow-up interview. The mother said she could not bring herself to take the bus to bring the boy to the clinic. He returned to his distant, small town to the care of his family physician who had neither a speech pathologist nor a psychiatrist to assist him in the resolution of the boy's condition.

In many patients referred to a voice clinic, the dysphonia has been present for a long time. This often leads to difficulty in determining the precise etiological factors in dysphonias of psychological origin. Not only do patients tend to forget some of the important anxiety-laden events surrounding the onset of their dysphonia, but the natural psychological adaptive mechanisms lead to the resolution of these conflicts with the passage of time. Otolaryngologists will be faced with the difficult situation of not being able to elicit the hard facts indicative of psychological conflicts which would enable them to make a positive psychiatric diagnosis. At the time of the consultation, the patient will seem relatively free of psychological conflict while still burdened with the dysphonia, the latter being the residue of the muscle misuse which arose during the earlier time of the acute psychological conflicts.

The habitual pattern of muscular misuse, irrespective of the pathogenesis of the symptom, persists in situations where the psychological conflicts seemed to have receded [9]. This situation strongly suggest that voice disorders should be evaluated as soon as possible after their onset for one to be able to identify the psychological etiological factors. Providing therapy is obviously also much more effective at this earlier time. It cannot be emphasised too strongly that, in the absence of organic structural change in the organs of phonation, the muscles of phonation are the final common path of all dysphonias of psychogenic origin and these will certainly persist if the misuse is not remedied.

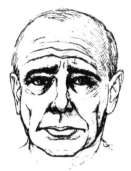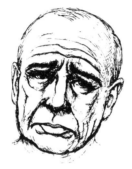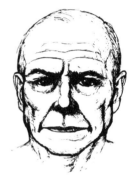

Figure 5.2 Faces showing (a) postures of chronic anxiety, and (b) suppressed impulses to cry or (c) express anger, are not uncommon in dysphonic patients.

As is mentioned in Chapter 6, facial expressions give clues to underlying emotional states (Figure 5.2). Long-standing failure to give expression to feelings of sadness or anger result in postural changes which, in some individuals, serve to sustain dysphonia. That being the case, it is not surprising that the abreaction of the suppressed emotion, resulting in the return to normal tonus of the muscles previously hypertonically or hypotonically restraining the overt expression of the feeling, often leads to marked improvement in the dysphonia.

Case 4

A 55-year-old accountant's weak, hoarse voice had responded quite well during speech therapy sessions, but the improvement was not sustained. He was a reserved man who had spoken but little of himself in the initial assessment by the laryngologist and the speech pathologist. He was referred to the psychiatrist because of the lack of progress in his speech therapy. At interview it emerged that he had been obliged to leave the small, country town where he had lived because of the behavior of his ex-wife which could only be described as very paranoid. Besides telephoning his employers, she had portrayed him to his three children in such terms that they had refused to speak to him. He thought that he dare not express directly to her any of the very considerable anger he felt for fear of the inevitable repercussions. In addition, he had reluctantly accepted his children's rejection of him without defending himself, as he felt their mother needed whatever support they were willing to give her. On reviewing these topics in subsequent sessions, the quality of his voice fluctuated considerably. He was encouraged to write what he would like to have said to his ex-wife, but dared not. In the privacy of his car parked on remote beaches he was encouraged to say angrily, even shout, his views. This he did conscientiously. There was steady improvement in the strength and quality of his voice. The gains he made in speech therapy now carried over into everyday use. Finally, he agreed to write and telephone his children to re-establish contact; his pent up feelings were further relieved when two of the three responded favourably.

When medical and laryngeal examination have established the absence of organic pathology affecting the vocal folds and the patient has received competent speech therapy, failure to improve should lead to a consultation between the otolaryngologist and the speech pathologist, the outcome of which might be re-examination by the former or consultation with an interested psychiatrist.

Case 5

A man of 50 years of age, who had developed baker's asthma necessitating the sale of his business, was referred after thorough examination to the speech pathologist for the treatment of falsetto voice; no improvement had resulted despite their diligent efforts. The psychiatrist was involved in the review by the otolaryngologist and speech pathologist and then interviewed the patient. With great reluctance and over lengthy interviews this stalwart individual added to the very sparse history he had been willing to give earlier. Not only was he being bankrupted by the failure of the purchaser of his bakery to pay him, but the Workers' Compensation Board would not recognize the validity of his asthma being work related. While he and his wife were contemplating the sale of their hard won home, the middle of his three teenaged daughters had run away from school and home with a drug pusher. He had not told his wife of his apprehension that his chest pains were due to heart disease. At this point the 'stiff Scottish upper lip' and determined smile gave way to muffled sobs; he was thoroughly ashamed of this unmanly behavior. Further questioning established the presence of a masked depressive disorder the treatment of which led to the resolution of the dysphonia. The return of his daughter, the improvement of his financial affairs and the absence of heart disease all played their part.

Similarly, where there is lack of motivation on the part of the patient to work in therapy, or secondary gain from the voice disorder is recognized, psychiatric consultation should be sought. A case exemplifying this has already been given.

A negative reaction to detectable improvement in voice is a further indication for a psychiatric referral, revealing as it does conflicting attitudes in the patient.

Case 6

One such case was that of a 27-year-old school teacher who had dysphonia of the spasmodic disorder type. During speech therapy sessions there would be substantial improvement in this patient's voice to which she responded by complaining that her throat hurt and she wasn't being helped at all; paradoxically, she was most reluctant to end the sessions. With some difficulty she was persuaded to accept psychiatric consultation. At interview she was most defensive, denying any psychological disability and emphasizing that her family could not accept the idea of her seeing a psychiatrist. It emerged that she was an extremely dependent young woman whose dysphonia had been precipitated by the principal of her school mocking her ethnic background and failing to praise her work despite the many opportunities she gave him to do so. She proved to be an extremely difficult case to manage psychiatrically. Consultations between the otolaryngologist, the speech pathologist, and the psychiatrist were gloomy affairs. She dismissed the psychiatrist on several occasions, would not do her speech therapy exercises and demanded that the otolaryngologist find some organic explanation for her disability. While she did become more independent and less demanding in her general functioning, and there was some improvement in her voice, it was only when she was given botulinum toxin injections that substantial improvement occurred.

The display of undue anxiety on the part of the patient during speech therapy may also require a referral, particularly when it disrupts the treatment. The patient mentioned previously certainly illustrated this point as well.

5.6 PREPARATION OF THE PATIENT FOR PSYCHIATRIC REFERRAL

As we are all only too aware, a number of patients regard the referral to a psychiatrist as tantamount to being offered an insult. That being the case, it is very important that the otolaryngologist or speech pathologist should prepare the patient carefully for the referral. He or she should portray the psychiatrist as a colleague interested in voice disorders and should refer to a close working relationship between them. A psychiatrist can be portrayed as more skilled in evaluating whether or not psychological factors are contributing to the voice disorder. Where appropriate, the patient can be assured that he or she is not seen as having a definitive psychiatric disorder. It is worthwhile to explain to the patient the role of precipitating psychological factors, muscle tension and anticipatory anxiety in the production of dysphonia. The interaction and additive effects of organic and psychological factors should also be reviewed as a part of the preparation.

5.7 PSYCHIATRIC TREATMENT

The dysphonic patient is more likely to be assisted if the attributes and interests of the psychiatrists include some, if not all, of the following [28].

There should be a willingness to engage in an active dialogue with the patient in order to establish a therapeutic alliance, rather than the maintenance of a rather silent and distant interviewing style. The psychoanalytical approach exemplified in the latter is particularly disconcerting to patients with voice disorders who usually have more than enough embarrassment about their speech for it to be emphasized by silence. Several patients whom we saw at the voice clinic had left previous psychiatric treatment for this very reason.

Willingness to become familiar with the physical findings on laryngoscopy, which require a close working relationship with the otolaryngologist, is highly desirable. This is frequently very helpful in diminishing any reluctance the patient has to communicate freely with the psychiatrist. This reluctance is also lessened if the psychiatrist works closely with the speech pathologist providing treatment. In taking the history it is particularly important for the psychiatrist to focus on each episode of voice dysfunction which the patient has experienced and the context in which it occurred; while this is important in itself it also facilitates rapport.

Competence in the use of hypnotic suggestion is also of value in a number of cases of dysphonias [26, 27]. A proper understanding of the misuse of voluntary musculature in patients with psychological conflicts enables the psychiatrist to collaborate more readily with both the speech pathologist and the otolaryngologist [1, 4, 5, 9]. Regrettably, psychiatrists with these attributes are relatively rare.

In summary, it is reasonable to expect that the psychiatrist will understand the terminology used by the laryngologist and the speech pathologist, with both of whom he will collaborate closely. Further, he or she should provide relevant consultation findings and focus his or her work with the patient on seeking to improve the voice disorder. Many of those psychiatrists who have psychoanalysis as their theoretical basis hold to the belief that removal of a symptom such as aphonia or dysphonia will inevitably lead to the manifestation of another symptom unless major work in conflict resolution is undertaken. This has not been our experience nor has it been found by those who work with behavior therapy. Where ongoing psychoactive medication or psychotherapy is required, it is to be expected that he or she will provide this in addition to the initial consultation.

References

1. Alexander, F.M. (1932) *The Use of the Self*, Methuen, London.
2. Allport, G.W. and Cantril, H. (1934) Judging personality from voice. *Journal of Social Psychology*, **5**, 37–554.
3. Aronson, A.E., Peterson, H.W. and Litin, E.M. (1966) Psychiatric symptomatology in functional dysphonia and aphonia. *Journal of Speech and Hearing Disorders*, **31**, 115–27.
4. Barlow, W. (1973) *The Alexander Principle*, Victor Gollancz, London.
5. Barlow, W. (1978) Anxiety and Muscle Tension, in *More Talk of Alexander* (ed. W. Barlow), Victor Gollanz, London.

6. Bridger, M.W.M. and Epstein, R. (1983) Functional voice disorders. A series of 109 patients. *Journal of Laryngology and Otology*, **97**, 1145–8.
7. Costanzo, F.S., Markel, N.N. and Costanzo, P.R. (1969) Voice quality profile and perceived emotion. *Journal of Counselling and Psychology*, **16**, 267–70.
8. Eriksen, C.W. (1965) Perceptual defence in *Psychopathology of Perception*, Proceedings of the 53rd Annual Meeting of the American Psychopathological Association, Grune and Stratton, New York, NY.
9. Feldenkrais, M. (1949) *Body and Mature Behaviour*, International University, New York, NY.
10. Friedhoff, A.J., Alpert, M. and Kurtzberg, R.L. (1962) An effect of emotion on voice. *Nature*, **193**, 357–8.
11. Gerritsma, E.J. (1991) An investigation into some personality characteristics of patients with psychogenic aphonia and dysphonia. *Folia Phoniatrica*, **43**, 13–20.
12. Gray, J. (1991) *Your Guide to the Alexander Technique*, London Victor Gollancz, London.
13. Guze, S.B. and Brown, D.L. (1962) Psychiatric disease and functional dysphonia and aphonia. *Archives of Otolaryngology*, **76**, 96–9.
14. House, A. and Andrews, H.B. (1987) The psychiatric and sound characteristics of patients with functional dysphonia. *Journal of Psychosomatic Research*, **31**, 483–90.
15. Hunt, R.G. and Lin, T.K. (1967) Accuracy of judgements of personal attributes from speech. *Journal of Personal and Social Psychology*, **6**, 450–3.
16. Hurwitz, T.A. (1989) Ideogenic neurological deficits. Conscious mechanisms in conversion symptoms. *Neuropsychiatry, Neuropsychology and Behavioral Neurology*, **1**, 301–8.
17. Ingals, E.F. (1890) Hysterical Aphonia. *Journal of the American Medical Association*, **XV**, 92–5.
18. Izard, C.E. (1977) *Human Emotions*. Plenum Press, New York, NY.
19. Johnson, A.F., Jacobson, B.H. and Renninger, M.S. (1990) Management of voice disorders. *Henry Ford Hospital Medical Journal*, **38**, 44–7.
20. Kinzl, J., Bierl, W. and Rauchegger, H. (1988) Functional aphonia. A conversion symptom as a defensive mechanism against anxiety. *Psychotherapy and Psychosomatics*, **49**, 31–6.
21. Kramer, E. (1963) Judgement of personal characteristics and emotions from nonverbal properties of speech. *Psychology Bulletin*, **60**, 408–20.
22. Mallory, E.B. and Miller, V.R. (1958) A possible basis for the association of voice characteristics and personality traits. *Speech Monographs*, **XXV**, 255–60.
23. Marxel, N.N., Meisels, M. and Houck, J.E. (1964) Judging personality from voice quality. *Journal of Abnormal and Social Psychology*, **69**, 458–63.
24. Markel, N.N. (1969) Relationship between voice-quality profiles and MMPI profiles in psychiatric patients. *Journal of Abnormal Psychology*, **74**, 61–6.
25. Matas, M. (1991) Psychogenic voice disorders: literature review and case report. *Canadian Journal of Psychiatry*, **36**, 363–5.
26. McCue, E.C. and McCue, P.A. (1988) Hypnosis in the elucidation of hysterical aphonia: a case report. *American Journal of Clinical Hypnosis*, **30**, 178–82.
27. Morsley, I.A. (1982) Hypnosis and self-hypnosis in the treatment of psychogenic dysphonia: a case report. *American Journal of Clinical Hypnosis*, **24**, 277–83.
28. Nichol, H., Morrison, M.D. and Rammage, L.A. (1993) Interdisciplinary approach to functional voice disorders: The psychiatrist's role. *Otolaryngology—Head and Neck Surgery*, **108**, 643–7.
29. Rossi, E.L. (1986) *The Psychobiology of Mind-body Healing*, Norton, New York, NY.
30. Rossi, E.L. and Cheek, D.B. (1988) *Mind-body Therapy*, Norton, New York, NY.
31. Salkovskis, P.M. (1989) Somatic problems, in Hawton, K., Salkovskis, P.M., Kirk, J. & Clark, D.M. (Eds.), *Cognitive Behaviour Therapy for Psychiatric Problems (eds K. Hawton, P.M. Salkovskis, J. Kim and D.M. Clark), A Practical Guide*, Oxford University Press, Oxford.
32. Sapir, S. and Aronson, A.E. (1987) Coexisting psychogenic and neurogenic dysphonia: a source of diagnostic confusion. *British Journal of Direct Communication*, **22**, 73–80.
33. Sifneos, P. (1973) The prevalence of alexithymic characteristics in psychosomatic patients. *Psychotherapentics and Psychosomatics*, **22**, 255–62.

6

Psychological and neurological interactions in dysphonia

Between the thought and the action lies a shadow, (T.S. Elliot)

6.1 INTERACTIONS AND DIAGNOSTIC DIRECTIONS

Dysphonia or 'bad voice' in the presence of a structurally normal larynx still presents a diagnostic challenge. Techniques such as videostroboscopy have demonstrated previously unrecognized structural problems, and new understanding of neurological conditions such as dystonia has increased our ability to manage more perplexing spasmodic voice disorders. But there are still many factors that seem to interact with each other in a confusing fashion.

Spasmodic dysphonia is a term that describes a vocal symptom, or a sign, depending on whether one is the speaker or listener. It is not a disease, but can be produced by several disease processes, which may either act alone or in combination with each other.

In order to make a clear, smooth tone that does not put undue stress on any part of the system, several requirements must be met: the lower respiratory tract must maintain a fairly steady airflow; the glottis must achieve an adducted position without overvalving; and the intrinsic and extrinsic laryngeal muscles must be appropriately balanced so they do not interfere with phonatory function. The degree of tension in the vibrating vocal folds is maintained in delicate balance by a complex neuromuscular system that is widely studied but still not completely understood. A few of the variables include:

- A tonus regulating center in the basal ganglia somewhere anterosuperior to the globus pallidus, and not too far from the seats of emotion in the hippocampus.
- A sensorimotor reflex arc originating in the laryngeal receptors that responds to glottic tightness, laryngo-esophageal mucosal irritation, and to subglottic airway pressure.

- A vagal pharyngo-laryngo-esophageal tube component in which glottic tightness may be part of reflux-related esophageal dysmotility.
- Emotionally induced glottic tension directly related to anxiety, depression, anger or sadness, particularly when the vocal expression of emotionally charged ideas is suppressed.
- Basic vocal technical skill, body habitus, and posture.

Adductor spasmodic dysphonia denotes a tense, strained, and often dysfluent vocal quality and effortful speech, due to hypervalving of the true vocal folds, and sometimes also the false vocal folds. The severity may vary from relatively mild voice breaks, to a spasm so severe that the patient must whisper in order to get words out at all. For some patients spasms occur more frequently on voiced phonemes when a vowel initiates the phrase, and on vowels in stressed syllables. For others, spasms seem more often to follow certain consonant sounds such as the plosives /p/, /t/ and /k/, which are produced with excessive intra-oral pressure. In the more severe cases, delayed voice onsets are often accompanied by extraneous muscle activity and grimacing that resemble secondary characteristics of stuttering.

In the absence of obvious mucosal disease or 'wild-eyed' psychopathology the tendency these days is to jump to the conclusion that the disorder is caused by a focal dystonia, due to degeneration in the basal ganglia. The assumption of this diagnosis may justify the use of botulinum toxin, the local injection of which produces most gratifying results. But, because of the nature of the chemo denervation, the results may be dramatic whether the cause of the dysphonia was neurological, i.e. a focal dystonia, or psychological. No doubt there are a number of patients with principally psychogenic dysphonias being maintained in good voice by regular injections of botulinum toxin. Inappropriate as this approach seems, it may assist the patient greatly when the social, emotional or vocal technical hurdles to recovery appear insurmountable. Remember that botulinum toxin is a Band-aid even for the patient with a neurological dystonia.

The list of ways that the mind can alter the voice seems endless: anxiety, with its accompanying aberrant respiratory and postural changes and generalized increase in muscular tone; conversion disorders; adjustment reactions; secondary gain; personality trait disturbances; dysthymic disorders; and depression to name a few. Add to this the laryngo-esophageal dysmotility associated with gastro-esophageal reflux, the inborn technical vocal athletic skill, and the possibility of a seemingly causative acute illness or 'organic trigger' and the stage is set for a puzzling factorial mosaic.

Physicians are trained to reach a diagnosis by collecting data about symptoms, signs and laboratory results and then deduce a most likely disease that can produce the presenting clinical profile, i.e. many clinical features with one cause. In evaluating the patient with a voice disorder it is necessary to consider that the inverse of the process is often true, that the one main symptom is caused by a group of ailments (Figure 6.1). Thus the patient who turns out to have a mild focal dystonia may be able to manage without botulinum toxin injections if his or her technical vocal skills are optimized, the depression and anxiety over conflicts at home or work are resolved, and any reflux or triggering illness is treated.

COMMON DIAGNOSTIC DIRECTION

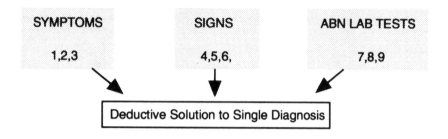

DIAGNOSTIC DIRECTION IN DYSPHONIA

ONE PRINCIPAL SYMPTOM - DYSPHONIA

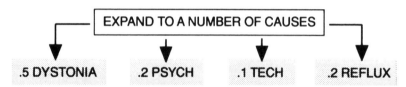

Figure 6.1 Diagnostic directions.

6.2 AN APPROACH TO DISENTANGLEMENT: SHIFT FACTORS IN DYSPHONIA

To begin this exercise, Figure 6.2 presents a graphic look at operant laryngeal muscle tone before considering therapeutically alterable patterns of voice use. It illustrates a hypothetical trace of muscle tension, with many individual people lined up along the abscissa, a point close to which represents normal tone. Since most people are normal, this line conceptually extends a great distance to the left. At the far right the muscle tone is very high as it would be in a person suffering from a focal dystonia. This degree of tension would produce a largely unalterable severe spasmodic dysphonia. The pathway from the low tension normal level towards the right side will likely follow a typical exponential curve.

If we now drop a line from midway up the curve down to the abscissa we may assume that those persons to the right of this point will have muscle tension that will produce symptoms.

But once a person's tension level has been set on the curve it can be shifted up or down (left or right) by a number of important adjustable shift factors.

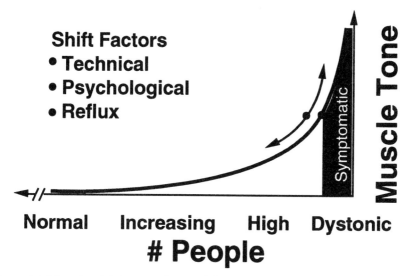

Figure 6.2 Interactive shift factors in functional dysphonias.

6.2.1 Vocal Technique

Proper use of musculoskeletal systems involved in voice production is an athletic skill that is more well developed in some individuals than in others. Figure 6.3 represents individual skill levels on a normal distribution curve, a biological standard. Most people who are in the middle of the curve do not react to the stresses of life by developing a voice problem. Similarly there are those few at one end of the range that have naturally excellent vocal technique so as to permit vocally athletic careers without being trained or coached. But at the other end are the 'vocal yokels' whose voice techniques are marginally adequate to get through the day, and with the addition of extra stresses they slip into dysphonic patterns.

A useful analogy is the game of golf. There are naturally good golfers who seem to play well right from the start and don't have to fuss too much with their posture or back swing. Although most of us with instruction and practice can make a decent showing, there are those who, for neither love nor money can get it right. Add a bad day at the office to your golf swing's peril.

6.2.2 Psychological State

Emotion is the intervening variable between psychological factors and the physically altered laryngeal muscle tone that actually produces the dysphonia. The most common relevant emotion is anxiety which itself has three sources; the threat of external danger, guilt arising from conscience, and apprehension about the strength of one's own emotions. Just as the face gives cues to the person's attitude and emotion, so does the voice.

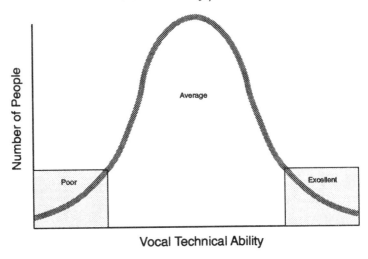

Figure 6.3 Vocal technique – a distribution of athletic skill.

Facial expressions, alterations in respiratory rhythm, and other postural changes that correspond to increases or decreases in dysphonia are useful indicators of significant psychological etiological factors. A patient may look anxious and the dysphonia may increase when he or she talks about a touchy subject, for example, the possible loss of a job, infidelity in a spouse, or serious illness in a child. Conversely, if a patient is distracted from topics laden with conflict and an animated exchange with the clinician takes place about a pleasant experience the patient has enjoyed, there is frequently a decrease in the dysphonia or the actual emergence of the patient's natural voice. In this case, the generalized muscle tension induced by the effects of arousal and anxiety have diminished, breathing will have become more natural, thus sustaining an even flow of air to maintain steady phonation.

A patient may or may not be aware of his or her impulse to verbalize certain ideas which are heavily charged with emotions of sadness, rage, or guilt, and the anxiety that accompanies suppression of these feelings. For one of our patients, shouting angrily at a handicapped child for his poor behavior was unthinkable, and episodes of aphonia and dysphonia resulted. For another, giving in to the impulse to cry about a dreadful loss would have threatened his self-percept of being strong, so he suppressed it by constricting the musculature of the larynx, neck and chest, since movement in these areas would have resulted in 'giving voice' to his grief.

6.2.3 Chronic gastro-esophageal reflux

For the purposes of this discussion the pharynx, larynx, and esophagus can be considered as a single, mucosa-lined muscular tube, all innervated through the vagus nerve. Reflux of acidic stomach contents into the esophagus is very common: an incidence of up to 10% of the population has been claimed. With constant acid irritation the lower esophagus becomes inflamed. This can be referred to the throat area, and result in awareness of a 'lump' or postnasal drip due to the common sensory nerve component. Since the acid irritation leads to esophageal dysmotility, muscle strain and laryngeal effort are often experienced due to muscles common to the esophagus and larynx, for example the cricopharyngeus. Persons with clinical reflux esophagitis or laryngitis must focus intently on learning and maintaining good vocal technique if they are to continue to have successful vocal careers. A reflux flare-up will make both the technical and the psychological aspects of voice use more difficult to manage.

When the clinician takes each etiological factor into consideration to formulate a problem description, it is less likely that the patient management plan will focus on a single issue at the expense of relevant others. The key is that each plan must be tailored individually to the patient need.

6.3 CLINICAL EXAMPLE

A 35-year-old female patient arrives in the office speaking with a voice that, in the examiner's experience, would be described as spasmodic. Unless this is a new presentation it is likely that the patient will have had numerous forays into the health care mill looking for help, and many therapies have been tried. But for now let us assume that this is a first visit for a disorder that began to emerge about six months ago and has only recently become a problem. The typical patterns emerge. Her voice is worse when she is talking on the telephone and in stressful encounters. It improves during laughter or singing and after a drink of alcohol. Other symptoms include the sense of a lump in the throat and the need to habitually clear it. Her voice is usually less effortful in the morning and this intensifies as the activities of the day progress. She has begun to miss time at work because of her voice problem and that is the real reason that she has come seeking help.

During the interview the following observations are made

- The clinician listens and watches for tremor. The presence of a tremor component strongly suggests that at least part of the diagnosis rests in the neurological sphere. Depending on the relative intensity of each component, the patient may be described as having a dystonia with tremor, or a benign essential tremor with spasmodic features. Take a careful look at the patient's handwriting for signs of tremor or writer's cramp.
- The clinician makes mental status observations. Is the patient direct in her descriptions and response to questions? Does she look you straight in the eye? Is there evidence of overt anxiety or suppressed anger, sadness or depression? Does the vocal quality vary with the topic being discussed? In the case of a psychogenically induced spasmodic dysphonia, the vocal tension may clearly increase when she is asked to describe her family, or her husband's occupation, and this change should prompt the clinician to probe a little deeper. This may lead to a detailed discussion of the patient's life and social situation to an extent that some clinicians are not accustomed. Nevertheless, this activity is worth pursuing, because

as one watches for tears, postural tension, frank anger or protective body language a glimpse of potential dysphonia-producing factors emerges. If the early bait is not taken and the emotional question remains unanswered then the clinician must consciously 'open some windows' with direct questions such as: 'How would you describe yourself on a scale of one to ten, where one is very relaxed and calm, and ten is tense or up-tight?' Then follow that question with: 'Are there things that tend to make you feel tense?' If yes, then: 'What?'

The otolaryngologist and speech pathologist are not generally trained in psychological counseling techniques but it is not unlikely that this is the first time that any health care professional has presented her with the opportunity to talk about these issues. Although some clinicians may be concerned about their ability to respond appropriately to this type of interchange it is usually the time constraint that cuts it short.

- The clinician observes technical voice use patterns.
- He or she determines the presence or absence of reflux symptomatology.

6.4 CASE STUDIES OF MIXED DYSPHONIA

As noted before, the single problem of a voice disorder frequently is caused by a group of etiological factors including:

- habitual postural misuse and faulty technique;
- chronic gastroesophageal reflux;
- psychological factors;
- an organic trigger, e.g. viral illness or injury;
- possible central tonus control problem.

Case 1

Joan Wilson is 37-years-old, she suffers from multiple sclerosis and she has a normal voice. Twelve years ago, at age 25, she consulted us in the voice clinic with a spasmodic sounding voice including the typical strained sound, with hyperadducted phonation breaks and obvious vocal effort. Joan seemed to present a normal personality and, although she dressed rather plainly, she did not seem to be depressed. The initial evaluation included assessment by the otolaryngologist and the speech language pathologist, following which she started a course of voice therapy. Joan's voice improved somewhat during two years of therapy but the improvement did not carry-over consistently to daily situations. Because of this she was referred to the psychiatrist who thought that there was still some psychological stress that required clarification.

Shortly thereafter Joan developed weakness in her legs and was diagnosed as having multiple sclerosis. Since there was an active debate going on at that time as to whether 'spastic dysphonia' was a neurological or a psychological condition, the clinic members took special interest in the diagnosis, and hypothesized that the voice disorder was an early symptom of the neurological disease. Thus, in our clinic she became a case example for the 'Yes, spastic dysphonia can be caused by neurological disease' side of the debate.

Two or three months later Joan told the psychiatrist of an event near the onset of her dysphonia. The night before she experienced an increase in her voice problems, (she was already hoarse because of a cold), her mother had informed her over the telephone about the accidental death of Joan's brother-in-law. Joan had previously described a choking feeling that she experienced as she received the news. (We already knew about this event, but not the additional ramifications.) It seems that Joan had long loved her brother-in-law. Needless to say her opportunities for fully expressing her grief were restricted. But once the significance of this emotional event was recognized, therapy could be directed at a specific cause and within a short time Joan's voice improved markedly. The effects of multiple sclerosis have progressed in other systems, but a follow-up after five years confirmed that her voice remained normal. Full recovery of normal voice occurred some months later, immediately after Joan had sobbed protractedly when she went to the funeral of a close friend.

Case 2

Susan Harris is a 46-year-old mother of four, who works as a college music instructor and leader of a children's choir. She came to the clinic complaining of two-year difficulty effecting the transition through the head–chest register during singing. Additionally, she felt both speaking and singing required excessive laryngeal and respiratory effort, fine pitch control was a problem, and the timbre (quality) of her singing voice had deteriorated. As a singing teacher herself she understood the dynamics involved but was unable to correct them even with the help of another singing coach.

Susan relayed that her career as an operatic singer and teacher had progressed well, but she had stopped most of her performance work about seven years ago in order to stay at home with her children. Two years previously she had resumed more intensive singing practice but experienced difficulty establishing her previous level of performance, despite concentrated work with an accomplished singing teacher. When she consulted us, she felt the problem was getting worse and that her speaking voice was taking great effort, even though to others it sounded normal. She had resumed teaching music in the public schools a few months previously, and feared she would not be able to continue if her speaking voice did not improve. She stated that a few sentences first thing in the morning felt more relaxed. She had given up on singing all together at this point, partly under the advice of her singing coach. Since Susan was known to have a small hiatal hernia she was started on an antireflux protocol plus ranitidine and domperidone, without immediate beneficial effect.

The ongoing team assessment included the laryngologist, speech pathologist, psychiatrist and the voice clinic singing teacher. The otolaryngologist was able to confirm a structurally normal larynx at rest, but careful review of the stroboscopic recording revealed an exaggerated posterior glottic chink (PGC) during periods of dysphonia, and asymmetrical phase and exaggerated PGC during register transitions. The speech pathologist found that Susan had several additional postural and technical misuses that might affect her speaking voice, and noted that she improved with diagnostic therapy designed to correct these misuses. The psychiatrist felt that she was mildly depressed and related this mainly to her home relationships. Her husband had transferred his business from eastern Canada and it had been her hope that the business would be successfully re-established here so that she would be able to devote time to her career as a vocal performer. Her husband had apparently been only marginally successful at his business ventures, which, in confidence, she stated was because he was lazy and incompetent. Since he was not sustaining the family financially she grudgingly continued to work at school as the principal breadwinner. The psychiatrist and speech pathologist both noted considerable variability in Susan's speaking voice with changes in topic. It was generally very breathy and dysfluent while she spoke of her family or career, but often improved for several sentences when she engaged in discussions on unrelated topics. The singing teacher noted several typical muscle misuses during register transitions and incoordinate breathing. The impression of the assessment team was that her voice problem was primarily related to an atmosphere of discouragement and repressed anger at her husband.

Susan started a voice therapy program and demonstrated improvement during structured vocal exercises, but no carry-over into her daily voice use activities, although she continued to practice the 'warm-up' protocol suggested. Although the psychiatrist felt Susan did not make any significant gains in psychotherapy, over the next few months her speaking voice improved and ceased to be a problem to her. She was still experiencing difficulty with her singing, however, and this became the focus of her concern once more. She consulted further with the singing teacher who found that techniques which reduced tension and improved vocal flexibility during vocal-eases, were not successfully carried over into her repertoire. We were now left wondering if there might be an element of focal dystonia. Not much has been written about the onset features of spasmodic dysphonia in the well-trained singer. It was felt that further laboratory analysis might help to sort this out.

A multichannel laryngeal EMG was made which revealed a consistent independent bilateral cricothyroid muscle spasm that began about 2 s after the beginning of phonation.

Susan continued to study intensively with the singing teacher and is now able to sing some of her previous repertoire with ease and satisfaction. Since Susan had revealed many possible sources of etiology for her dysphonia, and did not show immediate signs of improvement in association with any of the treatment plans, it is difficult to draw conclusions about the predisposing, precipitating, and perpetuating roles that neurological, psychological, technical and organic factors played in symptom formation and resolution. We would speculate that the focal laryngeal dystonia demonstrated with EMG assessment interacted with gastro-esophageal reflux, psychological stressors, and vocal technical errors to produce a variable hypertonicity in the larynx and subsequent incoordination for complex phonatory tasks. Since the purposes of speaking and singing may be quite different, these factors may have interacted in different ways for the two activities. We would like to believe that our therapy programs accounted for the gradual improvement in both Susan's speaking and singing voice, albeit somewhat after the fact.

Case 3

Lloyd Parsons is a silversmith and works in a small family business in his home with his wife as manager and book keeper. He came to the clinic with a voice very typical of adductor spasmodic dysphonia. It was readily demonstrated that he could maintain a normal voice when using techniques suggested by the speech pathologist, prior to resuming the dysphonia on leaving the clinic. Despite this finding, his speech symptoms were so typical of a laryngeal focal dystonia that we concluded that his disorder was of threshold severity only and he could have a normal voice while in direct therapy, and that any added stress pushed him aback across the threshold into dysphonia. Even though we knew that there was a degree of muscle misuse we were persuaded to offer him a botulinum injection. This produced the usual side effects and a much better voice for a couple of weeks, but the good results were very transitory so that a month after injection he was back to his dysphonic voice. After almost a year some psychological realities finally emerged. His father was a military man to whom jewelry was not a very satisfactory career for his son, and Lloyd was never able to stand up to his rather domineering dad. Lloyd then married an assertive, somewhat dominant woman and, lo and behold, he could not stand up to her either. It seems that losing his voice was as good a way to avoid confrontation as any. This relationship issue was very amenable to therapy and Lloyd's voice has remained normal now for over a year.

To summarize, the final common pathway in symptom formation for many dysphonias is misuse of the voluntary muscle systems that are employed for speech-breathing, phonation, articulation and resonance. Dysfunctional usage may be the result of a number of interacting factors, producing an etiological mosaic. Disentanglement of these factors may be a prerequisite to effective therapy.

7

Pediatric voice disorders: special considerations

7.1 DESCRIPTIONS, DEFINITIONS AND EPIDEMIOLOGY

Voice disorders in children differ from those in adults in several special aspects.

- Anatomically, the larynx is not only smaller, but also is structurally and functionally different.
- The types of disorders included in the differential diagnosis includes consideration of a wide range of congenital and genetic disorders.
- Voice pathology may occur in association with disorders of speech, language and other developmental disorders such that the mechanical ability to communicate may co-occur with, or be a manifestation of, disorders of the cognitive initiation of the vocalization.
- In the prelinguistic child, the clinician requires particular awareness of the relationship of voice with respiratory and feeding function as a localizing and diagnostic symptom in aerodigestive tract disorders.
- The limited cooperative ability of young children requires that the clinician take special care to select and administer evaluation and treatment techniques in the least invasive and frightening manner.
- The clinician must include the parents, family, or care-givers and educators as therapists.

In clinical practice dealing with communicative disorders, the overlap of language, speech, and voice disorders is frequent as many patients with developmental handicaps will present with difficulties in all areas.

In the mildest cases a disordered voice in childhood may be an indication of a focal laryngeal defect with minimal influence on the course of the patient's functioning in terms of medical health or communication. In other cases the abnormal voice may be a clue to a systemic disorder of congenital or acquired nature and can be a very important symptom in localizing a potentially life-threatening condition.

It is unlikely that the clinician seeing children with abnormal voices will be considering underlying malignant diseases, but potentially fatal lesions such as foreign body ingestion, acute inflammatory conditions, or histologically benign lesions such as mucoceles or papillomata may all have serious airway complications.

Regrettably, training of general pediatricians frequently does not emphasize abnormalities of voice quality as an important diagnostic symptom or localizing sign in the manner that auscultation (evaluation by listening) of cardiac sounds or focal neurological abnormalities might be evaluated.

Voice is regarded as a function of the larynx which has arisen as a late evolutionary process for communicative purposes. The primal function of the larynx is to provide an airway to the lungs, and a sphincteric valve to protect the lower respiratory tract. These functions are vital to the health and functioning of the individual. However, it is the secondary function of voiced language that provides a unique role in societal organization.

Most authors regard voice as having three perceptual dimensions; pitch, loudness, and quality. Wilson [21] notes that a normal voice should have a pleasing quality, proper balance of oral and nasal resonance, appropriate loudness, habitual pitch level suitable for the age, size, and sex of an individual, and appropriate voice inflections. Voice characteristics convey information not only related to the individual's laryngeal status, but also to social origins, emotional state, physique, age, and sex.

A voice disorder is noted to occur when these parameters are deviant. Wilson summarizes this impression by stating that if a voice is distracting or unpleasant, or if it interferes with the content of the communication, that a disorder is present. The disturbed voice quality may occur from laryngeal dysfunction and result in perceptual descriptions such as:

- 'hoarse', 'harsh', or 'breathy' laryngeal features;
- abnormal loudness;
- pitch inappropriate for age, size, or sex;
- inappropriate stress or intonation patterns.

In addition, laryngeal dysfunction is frequently associated with disturbances of balance between oral and nasal coupling, resulting from lesions affecting the velopharyngeal sphincter; obstruction in the nasopharynx; or glosso/pharyngeal hypertonicity. In this case, hypernasal or hyponasal resonance may contribute to voice quality perception.

The study of voice disorders in the pediatric population has usually been overshadowed by concerns related to language development and speech disorders. It is important that the clinician has a working understanding of the nonphonatory aspects of speech and language disorders so as to be able to distinguish between the voice disorder and other unrelated or interacting aspects of communication disorders. A brief review of these disorders serves to place pediatric voice disorders in the context of communication.

Language refers to a system of symbolic designations for objects, relationships and activities which are shared and learned. Language symbols serve to classify experiences for the purpose of communication. Oral language is transmitted vocally and received aurally, whereas writing, sign language and other nonvocal language systems are transmitted manually and received visually or through tactile sensation. Each language, whether oral or manual, has a grammar or syntax: a system of rules by which words or meaningful units are organized to make phrases and sentences. In oral languages, aspects of voice production, in particular stress and intonation, sometimes change the meaning or structure of a sentence. For example, if the voice rises in pitch at the end of the sentence: 'You are going' it conveys a question, whereas, if the pitch drops, it becomes a statement of fact, or even a demand.

Speech refers to the oral expression of language. Articulation is the motor function by which internal language is converted into sounds by movements of the lips, tongue, palate, pharynx, larynx, and respiratory system [3] for example rounding of the lips for /u/; closure/release of the lips for /p/; lowering of the velum for nasals /m/; /n/. Phonology is the pattern or system of rules by which the sounds are organized.

Disorders in the development of speech and language have been studied extensively [4, 9, 19]. These problems account for the major case load for therapists working with verbal communication problems with children and are usually the major source of parental concern when evaluation and intervention are sought.

Developmental language disorders are frequently associated with other disorders of development and intellectual function. Parameters of language skill form major components of test batteries used to assess intellectual function.

Speech development is a maturational learned process which occurs in stages over a four to six year period. The majority of speech disorders are articulation or phonological problems. Disordered or delayed articulation may be associated with organic lesions such as cerebral palsy, cleft palate, orofacial abnormality, dental problems, or neuromuscular disorders.

Stuttering represents a dysfluent speech pattern in which rhythm is interrupted by stoppage, prolongation, or repetition of sounds, words, or phrases. Etiology usually includes neuromuscular abnormalities, but stress and learned factors may contribute also.

Autism may be characterized by failure to develop appropriate language and social responsiveness as well as deficiency or distortion of speech. Stereotyped behaviors or echolalia may also occur in autistic children.

The incidence of speech, language, and voice disorders is higher in patients with mental retardation. Behavioral disorders are associated with higher incidence of speech and language disorders. Restless behaviors, attention deficit, or hyperactivity may occur in these patients.

Facial movements, throat-clearing, sniffing, and coughing may occur along with abnormal vocalizations known as 'tics' in patients with Gilles de la Tourette's syndrome (a neurological syndrome of uncertain etiology) [14].

Reliable estimates of the prevalence of voice disorders in children are not available, but estimates range from 5–25% in the school age population [16, 21].

7.2 NATURAL HISTORY OF VOICE AND VOCAL TRACT DEVELOPMENT

The pediatric larynx differs from the adult larynx in several respects which have important clinical implications.

The adult vocal folds in the female are 8–11.5 mm and 11–16 mm in the male. The newborn vocal folds are 6–8 mm. In the child the vocal processes of the arytenoids form a greater relative proportion of the glottis such that the membranous and cartilaginous parts of the vocal folds are approximately equal. The relatively larger area of the respiratory (posterior) glottis structures in infants serves important functions for deglutition and respiration: being designed to alternately valve rapidly and effectively to protect the airway during swallowing, and open rapidly for inspiration between swallows. Dejonckere [10] reports that, at birth, the lower border of the cricoid is located at level C_3 to C_4, but descends to the inferior level of C_5 at two years, mid C_6 at five years, and level of C_6 to C_7 at 15 years. At birth the thyroid and hyoid structures are contiguous, then separate craniocaudally. The alae of the thyroid cartilage form an angle of $110°$ at birth in the male and $120°$ in the female. The angle remains stable in the female with growth, but narrows to $90°$ in the male at puberty.

The hyoid is cartilaginous at birth, then begins to ossify at two years. The remaining cartilages ossify during adulthood.

The narrowest diameter of the pediatric airway is at the subglottic (cricoid) level [18].

In more than 50% of cases the infant epiglottis is omega-shaped in cross section, rather than a gentle curve as it appears in the adult. The infant's softer cartilages and lax supporting ligaments tend to collapse on inspiration. The subepithelial tissues are less dense and more vascular and are therefore more subject to inflammatory or post-traumatic edema.

The functional correlates of these differences are that the infant larynx appears more anterior and higher in the neck and is more difficult to intubate. The posterior subglottis bears the brunt of intubation injuries. The point of maximal vocal fold vibration occurs more anteriorly and may influence the site of nodule formation.

Minor changes in laryngeal soft tissue edema in the infant result in marked changes in the airflow resistance at the laryngeal level as airflow resistance is proportional to the inverse of the radius to the power four [8], for example: a 1 mm edematous swelling at the laryngeal level increases work of breathing by approximately 40%.

The histological development of the larynx is described in Chapter 10. The vocal fold structure is simpler in infancy. The mucosal layers are thick and there is no vocal ligament. The infant larynx has less type I muscle fibers which are responsible for slow, prolonged contraction. In contrast, a larger proportion of type II fibers may serve the infant's need for rapid glottic movement to allow rapid inspiration without aspiration during feeding.

The change in fiber populations with growth is thought to be correlated with increased refinement and variety of vocalization and the potential for training in later life. Corresponding increases in tongue strength and coordination occur to assist speech production. The vocal ligament differentiates in the preschool years and the vocal fold becomes two-layered at puberty. Throughout childhood the larynx grows in a relatively linear fashion provided that bodily growth follows normal patterns. In specific growth disorders such as achondroplasia, laryngeal size correlates better with patient weight rather than age.

The functional characteristics of laryngeal growth include a decrease in fundamental frequency as the larynx increases in size; and decrease in formant frequencies as the pharyngobuccal tube elongates. At birth the cry averages 500 Hz, then declines to 286.5 Hz at seven years, then 275.8 Hz at eight years, as reported by Dejonkere [10]. Average pitch range at one to two years is five semitones, then 14–19 semitones in 12-year-old boys, and 16–22 semitones in 12-year-old girls. During adolescence a rapid descent of fundamental frequency (up to an octave) typically occurs within the course of several months in males. The female voice declines an average of 2.4 semitones over the course of several years into early adulthood. The average f_0 for the female voice is 207 Hz and the male voice ranges from 120 to 130 Hz, until other changes occur in older age. In addition to the laryngeal changes noted, the vocal tract grows and changes shape dramatically from infancy to adulthood. The growth patterns of the vocal tract during puberty are different for males and females: the pharyngeal region increasing proportionally more in the male than female, compared to growth in the oral cavity. These structural developments alter the resonance characteristics in rather complicated ways. To simplify the effects, the frequency of vocal tract formants drops as the vocal tract grows larger, but shape changes also determine the frequency of individual vocal tract formants.

Emotive or communicative intent in the voice is recognized early in infancy. Specific cries for hunger, pain, comfort, pleasure or discomfort are recognized, particularly by the infant's mother or other experienced child care-givers. Loss of communicative variation in infant vocalization is recognized in infants deprived of social stimulation (P. Rodenberg, personal communication). There is a characteristic harsh, incessant, high-pitched, inconsolable quality to crying in newborns in withdrawal with neonatal abstinence syndrome after exposure *in utero* to opiate drugs (L. Salkeld, personal observation).

7.3 CAUSES OF VOICE DISORDERS IN CHILDREN

The differential diagnosis for voice disorders in children is extensive. Many of the potential causes are very rare and are beyond the scope of this text for discussion. The reader is referred to Maddern, Campbell and Stool [16] and Dejonckere [10] for detailed listings of etiologic lesions. These comprehensive analyses cluster causes accordingly to pathologic etiology, and include conditions such as disorders of resonance, and disorders in which involuntary (non-communicative) sound, such as stridor, emanates from the vocal tract.

The traditional classification scheme for voice disorders distinguishes between organic and psychological/muscle misuse etiologies. This approach, however may be misleading in its simplicity. As was described in Chapter 2, many 'organic' lesions including nodules, polyps, and ulcers may arise from muscle misuses that are due to habitual patterns with or without psychosociopathological conditions. In describing the nature of organic problems associated with voice dysfunction in children, it is valuable to differentiate 'primary' and 'secondary' organic disorders. The classification scheme for muscle misuse voice disorders outlined in Chapter 2 can then be applied to further describe the nature of muscle misuse voice disorders associated with secondary organic lesions, as well as those that are not associated with structural changes.

The most common etiology of voice disorders in children is vocal abuse and muscle misuse, and of this group vocal nodules predominate as the most likely secondary organic diagnosis of dysphonias in childhood. To the diagnostician it is the rarer causes that frequently provide the most challenge to investigate and treat, particularly when the voice is a clue to a systemic disorder or represents an indication that a threat to airway or vital functioning is present.

The most common pediatric laryngeal lesions are reviewed below.

7.3.1 Primary Organic Disorders

Recurrent respiratory papillomatosis is a relatively common disorder in which benign wart-like growths repeatedly grow in the larynx. The etiology is viral and potential acquisition from maternal genital papillomata is presumed to occur. The pediatric form of the condition recurs more aggressively and diffusely than in adults. Dissemination of the lesions to the distal tracheobronchial tree may occur and can be associated with a fatal outcome. The condition has been refractory to a wide range of treatments including surgical removal, fulgurization (heat destruction), cryotherapy (destruction by freezing), antiviral agents, radiation, and locally applied toxins. Currently, the best method of control to maintain airway patency is repeated treatments with carbon dioxide laser. Tracheotomy is associated with distal dissemination of disease and is to be avoided. Current research includes evaluation of immune system adjuncts such as interferon and use of phototherapy (light therapy). Spontaneous regression occurs with age in many cases. This condition forms a significant and frequently worrisome case load for pediatric laryngologists. Voice therapy has little role in treating this disorder, but may assist the child to optimize communication strategies when significant persistent hoarseness occurs following medical/surgical management.

Congenital malformations of the larynx include webs and aplasias. Aplastic conditions may be associated with malformations and fistulas involving the gastro-esophageal tract. The condition can be fatal at birth unless prompt recognition and airway bypass is undertaken. Laryngeal webs vary in thickness and extent. Tracheotomy is frequently required while surgery to divide the web is undertaken, according to Cohen [6]. Residual voice function is usually adequate for most speech communication situations, but may be enhanced by voice therapy to reduce inappropriate compensatory strategies and optimize and augment vocal loudness, pitch, and quality, once the child is old enough to cooperate in a rehabilitation program.

Laryngomalacia is the most common congenital laryngeal disorder. The condition is associated with nonvoluntary, noncommunicative respiratory noise known as stridor. It may be evident shortly after birth and persist for up to 12–18 months. The noise represents a loud inspiratory crowing related to airflow turbulence as the supraglottic structures (epiglottis, aryepiglottic folds, and arytenoids) tend to collapse with the inspired breath. The condition is a result of immaturity of cartilaginous development and is most evident in omega-shaped larynges. The great majority of cases require no therapy other than diagnosis of the condition and exclusion of other lesions. In a few cases the cartilaginous collapse may impair the airway and secondarily affect growth and feeding. Surgical resection of the collapsing tissue by epiglottopexy or laser vaporization may be needed.

Other laryngeal lesions such as subglottic stenosis or subglottic hemangioma have been of concern primarily for effects on respiration. Choice of therapy including endoscopic or open surgery may effect the ultimate outcome for voice function.

Vocal fold paralysis represents the second most common diagnosis of congenital laryngeal disorders. Grundfast reviews this condition extensively and describes the association with myelodysplasia and Arnold-Chiari malformation which is character-ized by caudal displacement of the cerebellum and brainstem into the cervical canal [13]. It is believed that 'stretching' of nerve rootlets occurs resulting in neurogenic laryngeal paralysis in patients with spina bifida and meningomyelocele. In cases where speech and language development may be threatened by impairment of vocal pitch, loudness, or quality, ongoing input from the speech-language pathologist is recommended. The SLP may need to provide augmentative communication options to ensure that the child is maintaining motivation to communicate, and receiving adequate feedback during verbal discourse.

Other congenital lesions associated with vocal fold paralysis include spastic and neuromuscular disorders including cerebral damage resulting in any combination of the cerebral palsy dysarthrias, and specific thoracic abnormalities including cardiac defects.

Acquired causes of vocal fold paralysis include nerve injury during birth or related to cardiac, thoracic, or neck surgery.

7.3.2 Secondary Organic Disorders

The most common voice disorders in children arise from vocal misuse and abuse. Vocal fold nodules represent the majority of the associated lesions and are identified in over 50% of children examined with voice disorders. The nodules are typically bilateral and occur at the usual point of maximum vocal fold vibration at the junction of the anterior and mid thirds of the membranous cords. Histologically, the lesions represent local fibrotic thickening of the vocal folds.

Precursor stages include local edema, then an organized inflammatory reaction before mature fibrosis develops [15]. Common observations in children with nodules are an exaggerated posterior glottic chink, and extralaryngeal muscle misuses and postural misuses typical of the laryngeal isometric seen in adults. These children may be observed to shout loudly during play, and may be participating in sporting or other activities where shouting and excessive voice use occurs. Throat-clearing, coughing, and abrupt glottic attacks may occur. The condition is more common in boys.

Green reviews psychobehavioral characteristics of children with vocal nodules [12]. They may be extrovert, aggressive, immature and may use voice as a method of asserting a role in the family or peer structure.

The etiology and management of nodules is discussed extensively in this text. A comprehensive review of nodules in children has been presented by Von Leden in

1985 [20]. He states that 'all current authorities concur that treatment of vocal nodules in children should be conservative' and cites that surgical ablation is unnecessary and potentially harmful as vocal fold injury may occur. He reports a favorable outcome with voice therapy and notes a spontaneous tendency toward symptom regression at puberty. If the causal factors or behaviors continue, the nodules tend to recur. Some guidelines for developing vocal rehabilitation programs for children are presented in Chapter 4.

Conversely Benjamin and Croxson [20] advocate surgical removal in specific conditions refractory to previous therapy in children older than eight years. The preconditions for surgery include long-standing symptoms, with social or educational compromise. He advocates forceps and scissor removal, preserving the underlying vocal ligament and vocalis muscle, rather than laser ablation.

Cases of previously diagnosed vocal nodules which have been refractory to treatment by voice therapy require re-evaluation. Mistaken diagnosis can occur when initial laryngeal examination has been difficult to attain.

Vocal fold polyps and contact ulcers occur occasionally in children. Posterior glottic pathology should raise the possibility of gastro-esophageal reflux or previous intubation injury.

7.3.3 Disorders of Muscle Misuse

Children may exhibit muscle misuse voice disorders in the absence of primary or secondary organic lesions. Psychopathological processes may play a role in symptom formation, including psychological states such as anxiety, and personality traits such as obsessional behaviors. In adolescence, adolescent transitional voice disorders (ATVD) may occur in males, and hysterical conversion disorders are seen more frequently in females. An interdisciplinary approach to assessment and management of individuals with these disorders has obvious advantages.

In addition to the many possible psychosocial influences on muscle function, muscle misuses may represent compensation for anatomical defects, such as cleft palate; or linguistic incompetence, such as language encoding difficulties or second language learning. In many cases, the voice disorder may not be treated directly in children with primary structural, phonological, or language disorders but, instead, initial focus may be placed on rehabilitation of general speech and language functions. Muscle hypertonicity in the larynx is a common manifestation of stuttering, and strategies for vocal relaxation and fluency can be incorporated into a speech management program.

7.4 APPLICATION OF TECHNOLOGICAL ADVANCES TO THE MANAGEMENT OF PEDIATRIC VOICE DISORDERS

The development of technological devices which allow for examination of children's vocal tracts without general anesthesia represents a great advance in the management of these patients.

Before the past two decades, the clinician was faced with the inevitable decision to recommend direct laryngoscopy under general anesthesia when indirect (mirror) laryngoscopy failed because of a child's age or limited cooperation. In selected cases in high-risk neonates, direct examination with physical restraint with or without topical anesthesia may have been advocated.

The development of fine-caliber (2 mm or less), flexible fiberoptic endoscopes has permitted minimally invasive examination of a wide range of patients with only topical anesthesia, or none at all. The coupling of videorecording has enhanced documentation for purposes of comparison with subsequent examination, parent and colleague education, medical and legal documentation, and visual feedback for patients during therapy.

Visualization of the child's larynx during vocalization gives better diagnostic information about function than can be obtained by observation during spontaneous respiration, but no phonation, under general anesthesia. This is particularly important in vocal fold paralysis which requires judgement and experience to assess [13].

The techniques for flexible fiberoptic nasopharyngolaryngoscopy are demonstrated in Figures 7.1–7.3. For infants, the traditional positioning places the child supine and requires one assistant or parent to immobilize the head and another to immobilize the body. Suctioning of pharyngeal secretions may be required via a catheter passed into the nares opposite to the endoscope.

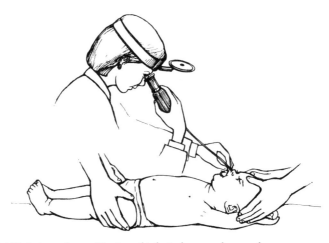

Figure 7.1 Techniques for positioning of infants for nasopharyngolaryngoscopy: supine.

Some parents of young infants prefer not to witness the examination, becoming anxious, tearful, or faint at the prospect. In this circumstance an alternative positioning is recommended, using one trained assistant and the parents waiting elsewhere. Stabilizing the infant in an upright position with trunk and head support allows good visualization with less pharyngeal stimulation and less reflux or retention of secretions.

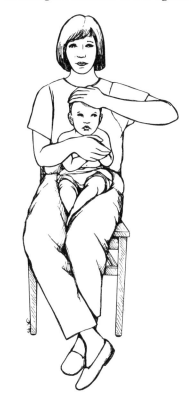

Figure 7.2 Sitting position for nasopharyngolaryngoscopy.

Occasionally airway, cardiovascular, or other conditions could compromise the safe conduct of the examination [13]. Significant airway compromise, cardiac anomaly, or arrhythmia history suggest that monitoring equipment, intravenous access, and resuscitation equipment be available.

The examination can be well tolerated in cooperative children as young as four to five years. The toddler to early preschool child remains the most difficult patient to evaluate, as safe restraint is difficult to maintain and cooperative maturity is not yet attained. These children and older patients with mental or behavioral disorders may still require general anesthesia for evaluation.

Chait and Lotz [5] describe the examination technique in detail in older children. These techniques are applicable for both velopharyngeal and laryngeal examination.

Whereas the flexible endoscopic examination in the adult may be undertaken by one clinician, it is very helpful in younger children to have a second trained 'team' member working in cooperation with the endoscopist, particularly when video equipment is to be operated during the examination. The endoscopist may wish to retain direct contact upon the child's face with the hand advancing the endoscope into the nose to discourage undesirable movement during examination. Effort should be made to create

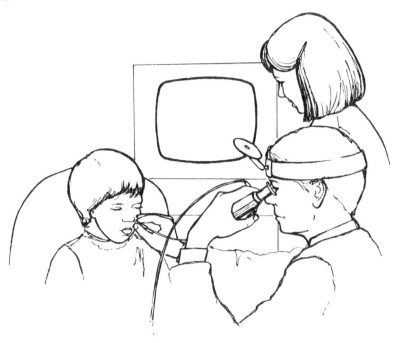

Figure 7.3 Positioning for endoscopist and speech-language pathologist during nasopharyngo-laryngoscopy with cooperative child.

a pleasant environment with a comfortable lounge-style chair, absence of 'frightening' medical equipment and 'white coat' clothing. The child can be encouraged by the prospect of 'being on television' and allowed to examine the endoscope and camera. During the preparation and examination, the child may be distracted by being offered a choice from a selection of small toys which may be taken home at the conclusion of the examination, or to work with a peg board or puzzle activity during the procedure.

Most examiners find that the effort to introduce topical anesthesia into the nose is rewarded by better cooperation for the examination. The least invasive techniques are best tolerated. Local anesthetic solution with or without vasoconstrictor solution is better applied by hand-held, low-pressure atomizer or dropper followed by sniffing, rather than high-pressure or machine-generated aerosols. Similarly, the introduction of anesthetic solution on drugstore style cotton-tipped applicators may be better tolerated than placing cotton pledglets with bayonet forceps or metal probes. Anaesthesia should include the middle meatus region for the purpose of velopharyngeal examination, as advancement of the endoscope along the nasal floor results in movement of the scope tip with velar elevation which distorts viewing of the velopharyngeal port area.

The use of stroboscopy in pediatric patients has been previously limited when the requirements of illumination necessitated the use of the optically superior, rigid fiberoptic telescopes. The introduction of stroboscopy coupled to flexible fiberoptic endoscopes has opened up new possibilities for the examination of children with vocal fold lesions.

The widespread commercialization of video games for children has familiarized young patients to seeing animated characters or other objects on computer screens which are responsive to their input. The use of specially designed hardware or computer programs for visual display feedback regarding pitch and loudness parameters, can be readily understood, even by preschool children.

7.5 VOICE DISORDERS IN SPECIFIC POPULATIONS

7.5.1 Hearing Impairment

The speech and voice characteristics of individuals with hearing impairment are abnormal because the ability to modulate production by auditory feedback is impaired.

It is traditional to regard children with congenital hearing loss or hearing loss acquired before two years of age as prelingual, and those acquiring impairment at an older age as postlingual. The former group have the most difficulty with control of pitch, volume, and loudness, resulting in inappropriate pitch, usually higher than that for individuals with normal hearing. Inappropriate loudness, (usually too loud), and minimal or inappropriate intonation, rhythm, and stress patterns are noted. In addition, abnormal tongue posturing may result in perception of a 'backed' oral resonance characteristic, which is also associated with articulatory/phonological distortions.

Wirz [22] discusses specific phonological changes and specific voice disorders. These changes are greatest in patients with the most severe and earliest hearing losses.

Voice qualities such as 'high-pitched', 'tense', 'flat', 'breathy', 'harsh', 'monotone', 'lack of rhythm' have been applied to describe the voices of hearing-impaired individuals. Postulated functional correlates include abnormal breathing patterns, increased laryngeal and supralaryngeal tension, restricted functional pitch range, and generation of high frequency turbulent noise in the larynx and vocal tract. Hypernasality is also reported in deaf speakers; however, this may reflect a perceptual abnormality induced by misarticulation of nasal phonemes rather than actual velopharyngeal incompetence. Deaf children may appear to use excessive effort in speech known as **over fortis**. This may reflect a compensation for poor pitch control, stress, and rhythm. Parameters assessed in speech and voice profiles show deaf speakers to have reduced tongue, jaw, and lip movement, reduced pitch and loudness range and variability, and generally increased pharyngeal and laryngeal tension. Acquired laryngeal pathology including nodules, edema, and polyps may arise secondary to the misuse patterns of vocalization.

Teachers of the hearing impaired are increasingly using visual display (biofeedback) techniques to enhance training, by providing information about the level and consistency of pitch, intensity and quality of voice, and the placement of articulators during speech. In addition, enhanced levels of acoustic amplification and tactile input (e.g. touching the larynx, feeling aspiration at the lips) may improve proprioception and articulatory accuracy.

In otolaryngology clinics, the parental complaint of poor speech development or loud voice is a frequent trigger for the request for hearing evaluation. Children with fluctuating mild hearing loss related to intermittent serous otitis media are noted to have periodic deterioration in acquisition of language and articulatory accuracy as well as loud speech.

7.5.2 Prematurity

The increasing survival of very premature infants, of less than 28 weeks gestation or under 1500 g or both, is associated with a population of children with special developmental needs.

Whitfield reports major handicaps in up to 10% of the patients including mental retardation, specific learning disabilities, seizures, visual disorders, hearing loss, neuromuscular disorders, and respiratory disorders (M. Whitfield, personal communication).

In addition to the cognitive language and articulatory disorders that may result from the neuromuscular and central processing problems, these children are at risk for laryngeal disorders related to prolonged ventilation. Extremely premature babies with bronchopulmonary dysplasia (delayed and inadequate lung development) may require weeks or months of ventilator support with chronic intubation.

The effects of red rubber endotracheal tubes in inducing glottic, subglottic, and even tracheal damage have been much reduced by the advance to polyvinyl chloride tubes. Tissue edema with diminished mucosal perfusion, edema, ulceration, then perichondritis and chondritis (cartilage inflammation) does still occur, particularly at the subglottic level where the posterior mucosa receives the major compressive and frictional effects. The induction of subglottic stenosis typically will occur in 1–2% of very premature babies in North American intensive care nurseries. These effects are aggravated when factors such as infection, poor tissue oxygenation, movement from seizures, or excessive mechanical movement by ventilator equipment are present.

The primary thrust of treatment for subglottic stenosis relates to the correction of the narrowed subglottic caliber and to removal of a tracheotomy cannula which is frequently required for airway management. During the past two decades the development of cricoid-split techniques and a range of laryngotracheoplasty procedures, in which the stenotic cricoid cartilage is divided, then augmented by the patient's own cartilage, have offered increasingly reliable hope of adequate re-establishment of the airway.

In the past, relatively little emphasis on subsequent voice function was given in comparison to the ultimate goal of airway patency. Increasing quality of photodocumentation does reveal gross and subtle changes relating to intubation including observation of glottic tongues of granulation tissue and subsequent furrows of tissue loss, as noted by Benjamin (personal communication). It is speculated that premature babies will be found to have perceptual and stroboscopic abnormalities when subsequent evaluation is applied. Vocal fold damage, diminished mobility by arytenoid fixation, and potential recurrent nerve paralysis may also occur secondary to the corrective surgery.

7.5.3 The Tracheotomized Child

In previous decades, the placement of a tracheostomy cannula (by the surgical procedure of tracheotomy) was usually a short-term intervention to bypass an inflammatory upper airway obstruction. The tube was removed when the condition resolved.

With developments in respiratory and ventilatory technology, temporary intubation rather than tracheotomy has become the usual treatment for short-term inflammatory conditions such as epiglottitis and croup. Long term tracheostomy is available for many patients with chronic respiratory failure who previously did not survive. These trends result in fewer patients with tracheotomy, but those who do require the procedure usually have complex long-term needs.

The development of expressive speech appears to be related to the ability to vocalize communication concepts, and inability to use vocal communication may impair development of cognitive aspects of speech and language in some children. Thus it is important that the voice-care team facilitate oral communication if possible for long-term tracheotomized children. Vocalization options include temporary occlusion of the tube during expiration by finger or flexion of the neck. Externally applied devices such as Passy-Muir valves have been well tolerated by children with good lung function. Electrolaryngeal speech has been accepted by some patients and has prompted creative strategies for its introduction (such as mimicking the child's father using his electric razor vibrating against the neck for shaving). Esophageal speech may be taught to certain older children with long-term tracheostomy. Total laryngectomy for laryngeal obstruction is seldom required in pediatric patients. In the rare instances of laryngectomy, however, the child may have access to the same methods of voice rehabilitation outlined in Chapter 4 for the adult laryngectomee population. Tracheo-esophageal puncture for voice restoration would not be considered until an individual has reached adult stature, as the stable positioning of the fistula is critical to long-term success of the procedure.

When oral communication is not possible, manual communication methods including signing, picture boards, or other electronic computer-assisted devices may be used [11].

7.6 DISORDERS OF NASAL RESONANCE

Nasal resonance may be regarded as a parameter of voice quality. Disorders of the velopharyngeal valving mechanism not only affect intelligibility by producing abnormal resonance quality, but also by inducing secondary changes in the function of the larynx for voice production and other compensations of speech production.

The nose is coupled to the respiratory system for the function of smell and for reasons of warming, filtering, and humidifying the inspired air. Involvement of the nose in modifying the quality of voiced communication is regarded as a relatively late function in evolutionary terms. Velopharyngeal closure serves to close off the nasal cavity during swallowing. Complex muscular interactions open the eustachian tube for middle ear ventilation. Closure is a sphincteric or valve action and comprises a component of velar elevation and a component of pharyngeal wall constriction.

7.6.1 Hypernasal Speech

In spoken English only the nasal phonemes /n/, /m/, /ŋ/, are spoken with the velopharyngeal (VP) valve open fairly wide. Inadequate closure of the VP valve for other sounds results in hypernasal resonance on vowel and vowel-like sounds, and nasal air escape ('emission') on consonant sounds with plosive-aspirate or fricative features. Associated features may include inappropriate muscle activity in the vocal tract; phoneme substitutions; dysphonia; and nasal or facial grimacing.

The disorder may range from 'assimilative' nasality (only sounds preceding or following nasal phonemes are hypernasal), to no ability to prevent direction of the air stream nasally. The overall effect can vary from a slightly abnormal resonance balance, often mistaken for a regional dialectal feature, to severely impaired speech intelligibility. In the most severe cases of velopharyngeal incompetence, individuals may also experience regurgitation (or reflux) of food and fluids into the nasal cavity. Examination of the velopharyngeal port with flexible fiberoptic nasopharyngolaryngoscopy can provide specific information regarding the nature of VP incompetence leading to hypernasal speech. The VP port is examined at rest, during vegetative activities such as swallowing, and during speech. Sound sequences with a high proportion of plosive-aspirate and fricative sounds tend to reveal the poor closure/coordination most dramatically because they require tight VP closure to achieve high intraoral pressure. Examples of test sounds and sentences used frequently include: /sasa . . ./; /papa . . ./; *Suzy at the sea*; *Pat the puppy*.

Hypernasality is readily confirmed diagnostically by the examiner alternately occluding and releasing the nares with his or her fingers while the patient speaks. In the case of mild or assimilative nasality, this test may be performed while the patient is repeating sentences or exercises with a high proportion of nasal phonemes /m/, /n/, /ŋ/; during sustained high vowels /i/, /u/ (which are associated with small oral opening, and thus are more readily perceived as hypernasal with VP incompetence); and sentences with a high proportion of high vowels. A cold mirror held under the nares during speech can be used to detect the presence of high levels of nasal airflow. Nasal flow during speech can be quantified with the same hardware and software used to measure phonatory airflow rates and volumes (Chapter 1), except a specially-designed nasal cone is used to receive the airflow, rather than the standard face mask covering both the nose and mouth. If the diagnostic equipment allows, oral and nasal flow rates may be measured simultaneously on separate channels to allow for a flow ratio to be derived. Otherwise the same speech task (same sentence, effort level, pitch, etc.) is recorded with the full mask, the nasal cone, and then the oral flow determined by subtracting the nasal from overall flow rates to derive an oral–nasal flow ratio.

Most usually, velopharyngeal incompetence in children is associated with cleft palate. Extensive discussion of the embryogenic disorder and subsequent variation in palatal clefting are beyond the scope of this text. Notwithstanding minor inter-racial variations in occurrence, approximately one child in 750 is born with cleft palate. Clefting may involve the secondary palate (soft palate and posterior portion of hard palate) and the primary palate (premaxillary portion) to varying degrees. When clefting of the alveolus occurs, there will be associated abnormalities of dentition, and when lip clefting occurs as well, there may be associated distortion of bilabial and labiodental sounds and abnormal structure to the anterior nose as well.

Other reasons for velopharyngeal incompetence include congenitally short palate, velar paralysis, associated with neurological defects of cranial nerve function, or post-traumatic scarring. An incomplete form of cleft palate may occur as a **submucous cleft palate** in which the typical findings include bifid uvula, a bony notch in the hard palate and a submucosal defect in muscular development of the soft palate. The mass of adenoidal tissue present in the nasopharynx serves to assist with closure of the VP valve. If adenoidectomy, which is specifically contraindicated in this condition, is inadvertently undertaken the predisposition to velopharyngeal incompetence becomes evident. Persistent hypernasality may occur following adenoidectomy in approximately one in 1500 children, even when no previously detected defect in palatal function was present. These cases may represent an occult form of submucous cleft that may be evident only as a muscular inadequacy as viewed by nasendoscopy, which may reveal a shallow depression on the nasal surface of the velum.

Transient hypernasality may occur in many patients following tonsillectomy with or without adenoidectomy which will be self-correcting within three to six months of the procedure.

McWilliams [17] reported the high incidence (84%) of vocal abnormalities in children with cleft palate. Most notable were vocal nodules. Other lesions included vocal fold hypertrophy, edema, posterior glottic chinks, and improper vocal fold approximation patterns. As these changes are deemed to be secondary to the velopharyngeal disorder, it is felt that primary therapy to improve voice quality will not be successful until the velopharyngeal disorder is corrected.

Milder cases of velopharyngeal incompetence may require speech therapy as the only therapy modality. The therapist may embark on a program to help the patient improve VP valving strength with speech and nonspeech exercises, in addition to helping the child increase the ratio of oral to nasal opening during speech, increase non-nasal articulatory dynamics, improve coordination between respiratory, phonatory and articulatory activities, alter speech rate and prosody (stress, intonation, and rhythm), and reduce compensatory articulatory strategies, such as the substitution of a glottal stop for oral stop articulation.

More severe cases may require pharyngoplasty surgery which may either introduce a flap of pharyngeal tissue to span the defect or attempt to create a sphincteric muscular valve.

The selection of the type of surgery is greatly assisted by radiological and nasendoscopy examination which defines the specific aspect of closure failure that is occurring. Other treatment modalities include augmenting the posterior pharyngeal wall with cartilage, other tissues or Teflon implant, or by the use of a prosthetic speech bulb (particularly in neurogenic disorders).

7.6.2 Hyponasal Speech

Hyponasal speech occurs when there is a reduction or absence of nasal airflow during the production of the phonemes /m/, /n/, /ŋ/ (ng). It usually results from structural changes causing anterior or posterior nasal airflow obstruction. To the untrained listener, this resonance abnormality may be occasionally confused with hypernasality, but simple occlusion of the nares during speech will not change the speech quality in this condition. Occasionally, complex combinations of hypo and hypernasal resonance occur if palatal fistulas are present, or if a cleft palate patient has anterior nasal obstruction.

Transient hyponasality occurs with upper respiratory infections or discrete episodes of allergic exposure. Chronic obstruction occurs with stenosis by bone or cartilage (such as choanal atresia) septal deviation, mucosal swelling such as allergic rhinitis, rhinosinusitis, or discrete neoplasms. The most common persistent cause in children is adenoidal hypertrophy which is typically most evident in the preschool and early school period.

Direct examination of the nose anteriorly and posteriorly (by mirror or endoscope) usually reveals the cause. Lateral soft tissue radiographs will show soft tissue masses in the nasopharynx. Rhinometry and nasometric evaluation of resonance on reading standard passages assist with diagnosis.

Speech therapy does not usually have much of a role in managing these resonance disorders. Treatment is usually medical or surgical, but nonintervention is frequently advised when regression of lymphoid tissue is anticipated.

7.7 THE YOUNG PERFORMER

The child or youth participating in dramatic or vocal performance requires special consideration. These individuals are comparable to young athletes performing to a high level of neuromuscular training. Traditional pedagogy has recommended that formal singing training not be commenced until the voice is mature, for fear of damaging the vocal mechanism. Other teachers, however, maintain that training may commence at any stage during maturation provided techniques of good vocal hygiene and appropriate repertoire are applied (B. Pullan, personal communication).

Young performers may experience acute muscle misuse voice disorders when the requirements of a cluster of performances rapidly raise the frequency and intensity of voice use to a degree well beyond their usual amount. These young vocalists frequently do not have the reserves of experience to perceive when strain is occurring and to modify their technique to eliminate it.

Frequently, the young performer is under great pressure to please parents and directors for monetary or social reasons and is conscious of competition and the need for early career enhancement. These pressures may be compounded by changes in sleep patterns, diet, and travel as well as adverse environments with respect to humidity, smoke, or other pollutants. Additionally, inevitable maturational changes in the voice may conflict with the performance role (e.g. the former boy soprano being encouraged to maintain his previous pitch range or quality) and in some circumstances the dramatic effects required for the performance (e.g. screaming, whispering) may require abusive vocalization techniques.

7.8 CLINICAL CASES

Case 1

A two-year-old child is noted to have progressive hoarseness over the course of one year. Medical attention is not sought until shortness of breath is noted. Prescribed antibiotic treatment produces no benefit. Direct laryngoscopy at a regional hospital is attempted. The patient becomes cyanotic at induction of general anesthesia and the procedure is abandoned without visualization of the glottis. The child is transferred by air ambulance to a provincial pediatric hospital. On arrival the child is noted to be aphonic with biphasic stridor and moderate costocervical indrawing.

Slow induction of general anesthesia by inhalation agents is undertaken by an experienced pediatric anesthesiologist.

Direct laryngoscopy reveals severe laryngeal papillomatosis such that 80% of the glottis is obstructed. Inspiratory–expiratory movement of partially pedunculated clusters of papillomata is noted. After biopsy and rapid debulking with cupped forceps the remaining papillomata are vaporized by carbon dioxide laser. Postoperatively, the voice quality improves dramatically and the airway obstruction resolves. Subsequently, the child requires repeated laser treatments at six-monthly intervals for modest papilloma regrowth. Good voice function is maintained.

Practice Point

The association of stridor and airway obstruction with dysphonia implies a serious obstructive lesion at the glottic level. Delayed diagnosis and intervention may place the child at severe risk.

Case 2

An 18-month-old child who has previously been well suddenly vomits and becomes agitated and short of breath while playing at home. At the local hospital a diagnosis of 'sudden severe croup' is made. The patient is unresponsive to inhaled racemic epinephrine (adrenaline) and systemic steroids. Urgent transfer to provincial pediatric hospital is arranged. Further interview with the parents reveals that the child has been unable to speak or cry since the sudden onset of symptoms. Direct laryngoscopy under general anesthesia reveals a spiral-shaped fragment of plastic wedged in the larynx. Severe associated swelling of the vocal folds is noted as well as minor lacerations and contusion. A minor chink at the anterior glottis remains patent. Following removal of the foreign body, the patient is intubated to allow resolution of edema. Antibiotic and steroid therapy is given. The parents recognize the foreign body as a component of a toy from the home.

Practice Point

Inclusion of questions about voice quality in history taking is of great importance in localizing pathology and suggesting etiology.

Case 3

An eight-year-old girl returns from a six month visit with relatives in another country. Her parents note that a change in her voice quality has occurred and her breathing is noisy at night. Relatives report that she was thought to have swallowed a piece of a razor blade while playing four months earlier, but medical consultation and a chest radiograph had revealed no abnormality. Newly ordered radiographs of the cervical area reveal an irregular metallic object in the subglottic trachea. Direct laryngoscopy reveals an irregular fragment of a stainless steel razor blade wedged vertically in the subglottic trachea.

Practice Point

If sudden changes in voice quality persist, full evaluation is required. Radiologic and clinical evaluation must be appropriate for the symptoms. When foreign body ingestion is suspected, evaluation should include the whole aerodigestive tract.

Case 4

A nine-year-old girl born with left unilateral cleft lip and cleft palate is reviewed by a multispecialty cleft disorders team. Past history includes extreme prematurity, hydrocephalous and ventriculoperitoneal shunting. Left vocal cord paralysis (neurogenic) has been diagnosed previously. Mild hearing loss, velopharyngeal incompetence, bucconasal fistula, malocclusion and a weak, breathy voice quality are noted. Management recommendations include alveolar bone grafting, Teflon injection to the paralysed vocal fold and subsequent speech therapy.

Practice Point

Surgery to restore anatomic competence to the vocal tract is frequently required before speech and voice therapy can be effective.

Case 5

A four-year-old girl has required prolonged hospitalization for severe asthma and chronic respiratory disease which is steroid dependent. She has suspected immune incompetence and has heptatocellular disease and ascites. Depressed affect is noted. Adenotonsillectomy had been performed for upper airway obstruction. She has a past history of recurrent otitis media and has a mild mixed bilateral hearing loss for which hearing aids have been prescribed. She has had chronic hoarseness with a breathy low-pitched voice and cushingoid facies. Previous laryngoscopy suggested edematous changes consistent with steroid use. Biphasic stridor of sudden and progressive onset occur. White fungating material is seen in the larynx and intubation is required. Subsequent culture grows *Candida*. Following extubation, carbon dioxide laser therapy is used to vaporize residual inflammatory swelling and intubation granulomata in the larynx. Hoarseness persists postoperatively. Voice pathology consultation is requested to improve communication skills. Psychology counselling is provided.

Practice Point
This case presents an example where multiple factors contribute to laryngeal pathology. Drug use, unusual infection and intubation change laryngeal structure. Hearing loss and abnormal respiratory function contribute to abnormal mechanisms of voice use. Multiple specialty cooperation is required for optimal management.

Case 6

A 14 year-old-boy is referred for voice evaluation because of teasing about a high-pitched, feminine voice quality. Peer comments include references to possible homosexuality. Pediatric endocrinological evaluation indicates normal pubertal growth with no evidence of hypogonadism. Laryngological examination shows evidence of normal male growth. Mild prognathism and high laryngeal position are noted. Vocal pitch range between 101 Hz and 290 Hz (typical for age and sex) is recorded, but a fronted resonance and articulation pattern are noted to convey an effeminate mannerism. Voice therapy and psychiatric evaluation are initiated and reveal no significant psychopathology. Good patient motivation is noted. Therapy is directed towards encouraging speech pitch less than 160 Hz and improving resonance quality.

Practice Point
This patient represents an adolescent transitional voice disorder. Consideration of psychiatric and developmental disorders is required.

References

1. Baumgartner, J.M., Ramig L.A. and Kuehn D.P. (1986) Voice disorders and stuttering in children, in *Clinical Pediatric Otolaryngology*, (eds. T.J. Balkany and N.R.T. Dashley) CV Mosby, St. Louis, MO.
2. Benjamin B. and Croxson G. (1987) Vocal nodules in children. *Annals of Otology, Rhinology and Laryngology*, **96**, 530–3.
3. Brain W.R. (1965) *Speech Disorders: Aphasia, Apraxia and Agnosia*, 2nd edn. Butterworths, London.
4. Casper, J.K. (1985) Disorders of speech and voice. *Pediatric Annals*, **14**, 220–9.
5. Chait D.H. and Lotz W.K. (1991) Successful pediatric examinations using nasendoscopy. *Laryngoscope*, **101**, 1016–18.
6. Cohen S.R. (1985) Congenital glottic webs in children. *Annals of Otology, Rhinology and Laryngology*, Supp. 121, 2–10.

7. Cohen S.R., Thompson J.W., Geller K.A. and Birns J.W. (1983) Voice change in the pediatric patient. *Annals of Otology, Rhinology and Laryngology*, **92**, 437–43.

8. Crone R.K. and O'Rourke P.P. (1986) Pediatric and neonatal intensive care, in *Anaesthesia*, Vol. 3, 2nd edn. (ed. R.D. Miller) Churchill Livingstone, New York.

9. Curlee R.F. and Shelton R.L. (1983) Disorders of articulation, voice and fluency, in *Pediatric Otolaryngology*, Vol. 2 (eds C.D. Bluestone and S.E. Stool), W.B. Saunders, Philadelphia.

10. Dejonckere P.H. (1984) Pathogenesis of voice disorders in childhood. *Acta Otorhinolaryngologica (Belgica)*, **38**, 307–14.

11. Fowler S.M., Simon B.M. and Handler S.D. (1985) Communication development in children, in *Tracheotomy*, (eds E.N. Myers, S.E. Stool and J.T. Johnson, Churchill Livingstone, New York.

12. Green G. (1989) Psychobehavioural characteristics of children with vocal nodules: WPBIC Ratings. *Journal of Speech and Hearing Disorders*, **54**, 306–12.

13. Grundfast K.M. and Harley E. (1989) Vocal fold paralysis. *Otolaryngology Clinics of North America*, **22**, 569–97.

14. Kozak F.K., Freeman R.D., Connolly J.E. and Riding K.H. (1989) Tourette syndrome and otolaryngology. *Journal of Otolaryngology*, **18**, 279–82.

15. Lancer J.M. (1988) Vocal fold nodules: A Review. *Clinical Otolaryngolory*, **13**, 43–51.

16. Maddern B.R., Campbell T.F. and Stool S. (1991) Pediatric voice disorders. *Otolaryngol Clinics of North America*, **24**, 1125–40.

17. McWilliams B.J. (1969) Diagnostic implications of vocal fold nodules in children with cleft palate. *Laryngoscope*, **79**, 2072–80.

18. Steward D.J. (1985) *Manual of Pediatric Anaesthesia*, 2nd edn, Churchill Livingstone, New York.

19. Van Dyke D.C. (1984) Speech and language disorders in children. *Annals of Family Practice*, **29**, 257–68.

20. Von Leden H. (1985) Vocal nodules in children. *Ear, Nose and Throat Journal*, **64**, 29–41.

21. Wilson D.K. (1979). *Voice Problems in Children*. 2nd edn, Williams & Wilkins, Baltimore.

22. Wirz S. (1992). The voice of the deaf, in *Voice Disorders and their Management*, 2nd edn, Singular, San Diego, (ed M. Fawcus), CA.

8

Voice disorders in the elderly

8.1 NATURE OF THE DISORDERS: AN OVERVIEW

While elderly patients may develop voice disorders from those etiological factors that affect all age groups, such as upper respiratory tract infections, they are also susceptible to changes that are related to getting or being old. Certain voice changes are a normal part of the aging process and should not be considered disordered, but it is important for the otolaryngologist and speech pathologist to recognize and understand these, in order to be in a position to help out when problems develop.

Some old men have thin, reedy voices that are higher in pitch than they used to be, and some women have voices that deepen with age. How far do these changes have to go before they cease to be normal? The answer usually rests with the individual patient's physical and psychological reaction to the changes, and the ease and effectiveness with which he or she is communicating daily. A change in 'vocal image' is often at the core of an individual's concern. When the older woman's voice is so low in pitch that she is addressed as 'sir' on the phone, she may consciously or unconsciously make muscular adjustments to raise the pitch. This tactic may work to a point, but soon the dysphonic voice resulting from muscle misuses associated with the attempted compensations are more of a problem than the natural changes causing the low pitch. Similarly, the old man with an easily tiring 'glottic fry' voice and bowed vocal folds may be suffering more from his subconscious attempt to drive the vocal pitch down to the male range as he is from the muscle atrophy, fragmented collagen, and weakened elastin of his larynx. Further, vital capacity of the lungs, chest wall structure, and elasticity of respiratory tissues change with age, and speech-breathing patterns may be affected by these changes [6, 24].

Vocal folds are made up largely of voluntary muscle, and voluntary muscles move them about. This neuromuscular system may become unbalanced by either psychological or neurological disease processes that are prevalent in the elderly. Neurological degenerative disorders, such as Parkinson's disease, impair vocal coordination, flexibility, and strength due to the same neuromuscular mechanisms affecting other voluntary movements, including articulation. Medical and surgical procedures that may be used to treat disorders common to the elderly, such as cardiovascular disease, may result in peripheral nerve damage, most commonly to the left recurrent laryngeal nerve disturbed during cardiac surgery, or intubation injuries in the larynx during general anaesthetic. Psychopathologies cause dysphonia via the final common pathway of muscle misuse. Most often, the phonatory production pattern observed is a product of both neurological and muscle misuse components, with the muscle misuse due to psychological or compensatory mechanisms, or both.

Finally, older people are more prone to cancers, and other systemic ailments that can play a part in forming dysphonia symptoms, including lower respiratory problems and gastroesophageal reflux disease.

In the physical examination of the elderly dysphonic patient one tends to focus on laryngeal function, but it is important to pay attention to other factors important to the speech chain, including hearing, general alertness and mental status, tremors or movement disorders, nonvocal speech problems such as dysarthria or abnormal resonance, dysphasia, and voice-related postural or musculoskeletal abnormalities. Transnasal fiberoptic laryngoscopy can be used to reveal abnormal laryngeal and pharyngeal postures and muscle activities during phonation. Stroboscopic laryngo-scopy in the elderly patient can help to differentiate between functional and structural bowing, and can demonstrate the reason for persistent dysphonia after laryngeal microsurgery by revealing stiffness, asymmetry, abnormal closure patterns, and other abnormal features of vibratory patterns.

To summarize, voice disorders affecting the elderly may have one or more of the following etiologies:

- changes due to normal aging;
- unsuccessful compensatory voice use;
- psychopathology;
- central or peripheral neurological disease;
- miscellaneous causes (organic disease, reflux, iatrogenic changes).

8.2 NORMAL EFFECTS OF AGING ON THE LARYNX

Studies of the laryngeal cartilage, muscle, connective tissue and mucosa have yielded a strong consensus about expected effects of normal aging. These include:

- ossification of laryngeal cartilages;
- atrophic changes in the lamina propria and muscle layers of the vocal folds, more pronounced in men, and often of concern to them because of increased pitch and a thin, reedy voice;
- edema and polypoid change in the superficial lamina propria, more pronounced in women, which may bother them if vocal pitch drops into the typical 'male' range; and
- vocal instability, including wobbling and tremolo.

These effects may be less evident in the presence of good physical conditioning.

Ossification of laryngeal cartilage continues until age 65 [17]. Islands of cartilage remain in the thyroid cartilage in the male, and preservation of cartilage exists in the upper portion of the female larynx. The cricoid may ossify almost completely [5]. The arytenoids undergo ossification of the body and muscular process, with the apex remaining cartilaginous. In general, the onset of ossification is later and less extensive in women, and the entire process is variable between individuals. There is nothing to suggest that this ossification process is related to laryngeal dysfunction except where changes occur in the crico-arytenoid joints. Kahn and Kahane [7] have shown that older articular surfaces undergo fibrillation and other changes in collagen fiber arrangement, as well as ossification that may limit the range of arytenoid excursion. When this leads to an inadequate posterior glottic closure, there may be a degree of air leakage which alters voice quality and intensity.

Connective tissue changes also show a sex difference. In the elderly man, the elastin fibers are fewer, fragmented, and clumped in groups. The number of collagen fibers is decreased with the remaining fibers being thinner, separate from each other, and more wavy. In women, the dense packing and linear relationship is preserved. The muscles of the larynx show general thinning and decreased fiber density, as well as fragmentation of the intermuscular septae [5, 17]. Sato and Tauchi [23] have shown a significant decrease in the number of both red and white muscle fibers with some increase in fiber volume after 50 years of age. After age 80 the changes are even more significant, but while increased fiber volume compensates, to some degree, for the loss of red fibers, the white fibers simply are reduced in number. Finally, there is a decrease in the number of fibroblasts seen in the conus elasticus. These changes are more prevalent in male than in female larynges [5, 17].

The changes tend to occur parallel to each other and in accompaniment with mucosal changes. The mucous membrane is thinned and atrophic. Mucous glands become atrophic and reduced in number, which probably has a drying effect. Metaplasia of the epithelium is seen. The underlying tissue may be subject to fatty infiltration, and the number of lymphatic channels is reduced [5, 12].

Laryngeal findings on physical examination are familiar to practising laryngologists. Honjo and Isshiki [4] found 39% of male and 47% of female larynges examined to have significant abnormalities. They also noted that 67% of these men had a glottic gap, a similar portion had atrophy, and 56% had edema. Women had significant edema in 74%, a glottic gap in 58%, and only 26% had atrophy. About one in 10 of each sex had vocal fold sulci.

A number of studies have looked at changes in speaking fundamental frequency with age. Mysak [15] compared middle-aged sons to their elderly fathers and discovered an increased f_0 in the older group. Hollien and Shipp [3] studied males from age 20 to 80 and found increased f_0 with age, with a saucer-shaped curve describing the relationship when younger subjects were included. They theorized that the vocal folds were thickest in the 40s and 50s and that the increasing fundamental frequency was secondary to thinning and stiffening of the vocal folds.

Studies of women's voices have shown that the vocal fundamental frequency becomes lower during aging [8, 14]. Another study suggested that this effect is less pronounced in well-trained singers [16]. The f_0 change is generally felt to be related to Reinke's edema and polypoid changes. Linville and Fisher [8, 9], however, have shown that the first formant frequency is also lowered for both phonated and whispered voice, thus suggesting that both phonatory and resonance features play a role in defining age characteristics of women's voices.

There is less agreement in findings regarding pitch range. McGlone and Hollien [13] determined that pitch range was largely preserved in elderly women, whereas Ptacek [18] found a loss of the high-tone production in both sexes, and Luchsinger's study supported this [12]. Aronsen's larger study supported the preservation of pitch range in both sexes [1]. Peppard [16] found that elderly trained singers maintained a wider pitch range than elderly nonsingers. Methodology differences in each series may be responsible for the apparently conflicting results.

Ramig [19, 20] has shown that fundamental frequency changes and quality differences, as manifested by maximum phonation time and pitch range, and jitter and shimmer values respectively, may be caused as much or more by general physical condition as by chronological age in men. Physical conditioning is also implicated as a factor determining certain voice characteristics of postmenopausal women. Lowery [11] noted that older women who engaged in regular aerobic exercise had lower stroboscopic ratings of vocal fold aperiodicity, asymmetry, and supraglottic constriction patterns, and were rated as having relatively younger voices for their ages than were women who were not aerobic exercisers. Exercises that are designed specifically to maintain good vocal conditioning, i.e. those used by trained singers, may contribute further to minimizing aging effects on voice function. According to Peppard [16], voice training may have an effect of maintaining lower perturbation, noise levels, and aberrant acoustic-perceptual features in voices of older women, which may be due to greater flexibility, regularity and symmetry of vocal fold movements, greater glottic efficiency, and lower degress of supraglottic activity in senescent trained singers.

Other age-related voice changes include a wobbling of the voice, attributed to irregular respirations, and the tremulous voice or **senile tremolo**. Some of these changes can be demonstrated as increased fundamental frequency standard deviation and altered jitter scores [10].

In summary, it seems that there are two general altered states in the larynx that develop with aging. One state is a thickened, chronically edematous larynx, with phonation in the lower part of the voice range and a husky or muffled timbre (mostly women). Atrophic changes predominate in the other state. These patients develop a squeaky voice from using the upper end of their range, and the vocal timbre is thin and reedy (mostly men).

8.3 DISORDERS DUE TO ATTEMPTS TO COMPENSATE FOR NORMAL AGING PROCESSES

As already described, the aging process in the male larynx involves muscle atrophy and loss of elasticity. The normal voice effect is increased pitch and 'thinning' of the vocal tone. Attempts to compensate for these changes usually result in glottic fry phonation, increased laryngeal effort and, subsequently, rapid vocal fatigue. Indirect laryngoscopy reveals apparent shortening and bowing of the true vocal folds. The vocal folds may adduct more efficiently if lengthening can be achieved by higher-pitched phonation. If women also experienced pitch increase in later life, it would not be perceived as a problem, since the higher pitch would be considered socially acceptable and therefore not likely to result in a functional misuse because of unsuccessful compensation.

Some degree of polypoid degeneration and Reinke's edema has been described as developing in the vocal folds of older persons. Distinct from the atrophic changes already described, these polypoid thickenings are more noticeable in women since they result naturally in a pitch drop. This more masculine-sounding voice, which occurs mainly in women who have smoked for many years, is socially unacceptable to some patients, although perhaps less so in the past few decades as women are socially condoned in using lower-pitched voices. For those older women who attempt to correct the pitch change, the most common compensatory misuse is lateral squeezing of the larynx in an attempt to increase vocal pitch. This may be quite dramatic to the stage of ventricular band dysphonia, or may be associated only with a mild false adduction and an apparent increased tension in the true folds with increased vocal effort. Phonation becomes easier and clearer when the patient is encouraged to allow the vocal tone to drop to a more natural range that is consistent with the polypoid change.

To summarize, the usual compensatory misuses are as follows:

Men

- Attempts to drop pitch
- Gravelly, weak, glottic fry
- Easy fatigue

Women

- Attempts to raise pitch
- Squeezed, strained
- Effortful voice
- Variable ventricular band adduction

8.4 PSYCHOGENIC VOICE DISORDERS IN THE ELDERLY

The elderly are subject to the same psychopathological processes that affect all age groups and these have already been covered extensively in Chapter 5. In older patients, loneliness or separation from family frequently lead to depression and tension. There is, logically, considerable overlap between those patients who have dysphonia as a result of attempting to compensate for age-related changes and those patients who have purely psychogenic dysphonias. Consequently, when evaluating an elderly patient with a voice disorder characterized by muscle misuse, it may be difficult for the clinician to determine just how much of the etiology is psychogenic and how much is compensatory misuse. The relative ease with which changes can be elicited during a voice therapy program may help sort this out.

8.5 VOICE DISORDERS AND NEUROLOGICAL DISEASE

Neurological diseases tend to occur more commonly in the elderly and, as would be expected, associated voice difficulties present from time to time. There are a number of neurological diseases in which the voice may be abnormal, but these seldom pose a diagnostic problem for the otolaryngologist since they are rarely the presenting symptom. Examples include stroke, amyotrophic lateral sclerosis, pseudobulbar palsy, and so on. Dysphonia, however, may be the presenting symptom of a neurological disorder. Essential tremor, often readily identified in the hands, may also exist as a vocal tremor that causes frequency or intensity fluctuations at a rate of 4–12 Hz. Tremor of the voice is consistent for most phonatory tasks, although it is usually most evident during sustained phonation of a single vowel in the middle to lower end of the pitch range and is often intensified with efforts to increase loudness. Many individuals compensate for the neurological instability by hyperadducting the larynx, and 'splinting' it with jaw, tongue, and neck tension. The result is low-pitched phonation that is dysfluent and harsh, and may be accompanied by phonation breaks similar to those heard with nontremor spasmodic dysphonia.

A weak, monotone, breathy voice with loss of expression and disturbed rhythm may be a presenting symptom of Parkinson's disease [1, 2]. Dyscoordinate or 'shallow' speech-breathing, and reduced dynamics of the laryngeal and articulatory muscles due to rigidity account for these prosody, intensity, and voice quality changes. The problem can be alleviated somewhat with antiparkinsonian drugs and voice therapy [21, 22].

Focal dystonias in the head and neck can result in prolonged muscle spasms leading to blepharospasm, oral mandibular dystonia, spasmodic torticollis or laryngeal dystonia. As with the other focal dystonias, these tend to be refractory to most forms of treatment except symptomatic chemodenervation. Botulinum toxin injections have been successful in reducing these symptoms in older patients with adductor spasmodic dysphonias. Although very effective for relieving spasm, it is less so for essential tremor. In spite of this, many older patients with combined tremor and spasm get significant relief from the injections.

8.6 MISCELLANEOUS CAUSES OF DYSPHONIA IN THE ELDERLY

Cancers of the larynx, and other tumors, may produce voice changes, and although these disorders make up an important segment of the elderly dysphonic population, they have been discussed elsewhere. The same may be said for the voice symptoms accompanying gastro-esophageal reflux disease.

Laryngeal trauma in this age group is more often than not iatrogenic. An example that is too common is the elderly female patient with mild or moderate polypoidal degeneration or Reinke's edema who undergoes removal of the polypoid tissue only to develop much more severe dysphonia because of scarring of the surface of the vocal fold and subsequent tethering of the overlying mucosa. The resultant stiffness and loss of the mucosal wave is clearly visible with stroboscopy. Once established, this condition may produce long-standing dysphonia for which most treatments are ineffective.

8.7 TREATMENT OF VOICE DISORDERS IN THE ELDERLY

Most age-related voice changes result from natural physiological degenerative processes. So how should patients for whom these changes are a problem be treated? Should we coax them into accepting their 'old voices' and help them reduce their compensatory muscle misuses and maximize vocal performance? Should we offer dissection or suction removal of submucosal tissue of Reinke's edema or early polypoidal degeneration? Should we simply counsel them regarding the interacting factors resulting in voice change and let nature take its course? The treatment plan clearly depends on a team decision, with the patient leading the team. We will outline the primary aspects of the treatment program.

8.7.1 Counselling

Often the elderly patient needs only to be reassured that the changes they are detecting in their voice do not represent any life-threatening illness. In some cases, helping them to understand why things are changing as they are is all the treatment that is needed.

8.7.2 Voice Therapy

Therapy for voice disorders in the elderly is frequently focused on reducing the muscular misuses that accompany attempts by the patient to compensate for the changes that have occurred. The therapy program may be directed towards encouraging the upward adjustment of vocal pitch in the elderly man with thinning vocal folds, coupled with any necessary alterations of respiratory support and resonance. In women, it may consist of encouraging them to accept a deeper vocal pitch and to develop an easier, more relaxed style of laryngeal muscle use. Therapy programs for elderly patients with neurological disease that lead to weakness or incoordination, or both, may be comprehensive and intensive. Goals of therapy exercises may include increases in respiratory support, vocal fold adduction, sustained phonations, vocal steadiness, pitch range, resonance sensations, and articulatory precision. As with many problems of incoordination, training in reducing speaking rate may have a generalized, positive effect on vocal production and speech intelligibility.

8.7.3 Psychological Management

Counseling by the laryngologist and the speech pathologist, and the direct voice therapy program, make up a major portion of the management of psychological components of the dysphonia. The reassurance and attentive care that patients receive during this process cannot help but have positive therapeutic effects. In some cases, however, where associated anxiety or depression, or both, is a major causative factor in dysphonia, management may be more difficult without assistance from a psychologist or psychiatrist.

Sometimes voice disorders in elderly people reflect their general social situations. They may find themselves living alone, with little opportunity to use their voices except on the telephone. In persons for whom this lifestyle reflects a major change or is clearly undesirable to them, we encourage and support them in altering this social situation to permit more frequent, direct voice use and better mental health.

8.7.4 Medical Management

The nature of direct medical management of dysphonia depends on the cause and may involve treating neurological disorders. The point has already been made about managing problems of chronic gastro-esophageal reflux when associated with a dysphonia, and this is often a most useful medical adjunct to treatment.

8.7.5 Surgical Management

Conservatism in surgery should be the general rule when managing elderly patients with voice disorders, particularly when treating patients with polypoidal degeneration. If the voice problem is of a severity to warrant surgical treatment, and if altering voice use through a therapy program has not been successful, then reduction in the amount of polypoidal degeneration may be warranted. This entails removal of the Reinke's space edema tissue only, with maintenance of the epithelial cover. It can be accomplished by making an incision laterally along the superior aspect of the vocal fold and reflecting the mucosal flap medially toward the free margin. Cup forceps, alligator forceps, or suction can then be used to ease the gelatinous polypoidal tissue away from the underlying deep layers of the lamina propria. Mucosa can then be draped back over the vocal fold. Fibrin glues such as Tisseel can be helpful in keeping the mucosa in place.

The treatment of voice disorders associated with scarring and mucosal tethering following vocal fold stripping can be difficult. These dysphonias are often unresponsive to voice therapy, and injection of the folds with substances such as teflon is generally not helpful. The use of collagen to inject the vocal folds submucosally is still being evaluated, but may hold some promise.

References

1. Aronson, A.E. (1985) *Clinical Voice Disorders: an Interdisciplinary Approach.* Thieme-Stratton New York.
2. Critchley, B.M.R. (1981) Speech disorders of parkinsonism: a review *Journal of Neurology, Neurosurgery and Psychiatry,* **44**, 751–8.
3. Hollien H. and Shipp T. (1972) Speaking fundamental frequency and chronologic age in males. *Journal of Speech and Hearing Research,* **15**, 155–9.
4. Honjo I. and Isshiki N. (1979) *Laryngoscopic and Vocal Characteristics of Aged Persons.* Kansai Medical University, Osaka.
5. Kahane J.C. (1983) A survey of age-related changes in the connective tissues of the human

adult laryns, in *Vocal Fold Physiology (eds) D.M. Bless and J.H. Abbs.* College-Hill San Diego, CA.

6. Kahane J.C. (1981) Anatomic and physiologic changes in the aging peripheral speech mechanism, in *Aging: Communication Processes and Disorders.* Grune & Stratton, New York.

7. Kahn A.R. and Kahane J.C. (1986) India ink pinprick assessment of age-related changes in the crico-arytenoid joint (CAJ) articular surfaces. *Journal of Speech and Hearing Research,* **4,** 536–43.

8. Linville S.E. and Fisher H.B. (1985) Acoustic characteristics of perceived versus actual vocal age in controlled phonation by adult females. *Journal of the Acoustic Society of America,* **78,** 40–8.

9. Linville S.E. and Fisher H.B. (1985) Acoustic characteristics of women's voices with advancing age. *Journal of Gerontology,* **3,** 324–30.

10. Linville S.E. and Korabic E.W. (1987) Fundamental frequency stability characteristics of elderly women's voices. *Journal of the Acoustic Society of America,* **4,** 1196–9.

11. Lowery D.B. (1993) Aerobic exercise effects on the post-menopausal voice. Doctoral Dissertation, University of Wisconsin-Madison.

12. Luchsinger R. and Arnold G. (1965) Vocal involution or senescence of the voice, in *Voice-Speech-Language.* Wadsworth, Belmont, C.A.

13. McGlone R. and Hollien H. (1963) Vocal pitch characteristics of aged women. *Journal of Speech and Hearing Research,* **6,** 164–70.

14. Morgan E.E. and Rastatter M. (1986). Variability of voice fundamental frequency in elderly female speakers. *Perception and Motor Skills,* **1,** 215–18.

15. Mysak E.D. (1959). Pitch and duration characteristics of older males. *Journal of Speech and Hearing Research,* **2,** 46–54.

16. Peppard R.C. (1990) Effects of aging on selected vocal characteristics of female singers and non-singers. Doctoral dissertation, University of Wisconsin-Madison.

17. Pressman J.J. and Keleman G. (1955) Physiology of the larynx. *Physiology Reviews,* **35,** 513–15.

18. Ptacek P., Sander E.K., Malone W.H. and Jackson C.C.R. (1966) Phonatory and related changes with advanced age. *Journal of Speech and Hearing Research,* **9,** 353–60.

19. Ramig L.A. and Ringel R.L. (1983) Effects of physiological aging on selected acoustic characteristics of voice. *Journal of Speech and Hearing Research,* **1,** 22–30.

20. Ramig L.A. (1983) Effects of physiological aging on vowel spectral noise. *Journal of Gerontology,* **2,** 223–5.

21. Ramig L.A., Horii Y and Bonitati C (1991) The efficacy of voice therapy for patients with parkinson's disease. *National Centre for Voice and Speech Status Progress Report,* University of Iowa, Iowa City, IO, pp. 61–86.

22. Ramig L.A. and Scherer R.C. (1992) Speech therapy for neurologic disorders of the larynx, in *Neurologic Disorders of the Larynx* (eds A. Blitzer *et al.*). Thieme Medical, New York, pp. 163–81.

23. Sato T. and Tauchi H. (1982) Age changes in human vocal muscle. *Mechanisms of Ageing Development,* **18,** 67–74.

24. Sperry E.E. and Klich R.J. (1992) Speech-breathing in senescent and younger women during oral reading. *Journal of Speech and Hearing Research,* **35,** 1246–55.

9

The singing teacher in the voice clinic

The singing teacher is a valuable member of the voice care team and, when interacting in a patient evaluation with the laryngologist and speech pathologist, can provide extremely useful insights, particularly with the detection of errors in vocal production. The singing teacher may also provide guidance towards finding techniques that reduce vocal misuse and work directly with the singer to rebuild the voice. This chapter presents an approach to this process that has worked well in our clinic. Chapter 11 discusses the art and science of training the singing voice from a more direct pedagogical aspect.

9.1 DETECTING TECHNICAL ERRORS IN VOCAL PRODUCTION

9.1.1 Appearance

The first and, in some ways, the most reliable method of detecting errors in vocal production is observation. When something is going wrong in singing, it is invariably the result of mechanical misalignment or misuse and nearly always shows in the posture, body language, and face of the singer.

Head and neck

The posture of the head and neck is a critical factor in body alignment, and any misalignment not only provides a visual clue to faulty technique but also is often the cause of it. The head is often held stiffly on a neck that is either hyperflexed or hyperextended.

The chin can either be tucked in with the head pulled down or thrust forward with the head tilted upward. Sometimes the head is held at an angle to the left or right side, or it may be observed to shake (often in time to a forced vibrato).

Hypertonicity can cause the muscles and even the blood vessels in the neck to stand out in relief.

Spine, knees, and body balance

The body is often seen to be held rigidly with braced knees and a 'sway back'. Balance may be poor due to unnatural weight distribution: either too far forward or back in the stance. The body begins to sway halfway through a phrase so the weight distribution is constantly changing.

Shoulders and chest

The shoulders may be held tensely so the chest is constricted, particularly on longer phrases. As the chest collapses during a sung phrase, the shoulders may fall forward. The opposite action can also be observed where shoulders are pulled back behind a firmly raised chest like a miltary 'at attention'.

Arms and hands

The arms may be held rigidly with the elbows out and away from the body, assisting in depressing the chest and tensing the shoulders. The arm tension often leads to tense involuntary hand gestures during a phrase or song, or to the hands being rigidly clasped in front or behind the body.

Face and lips

The face will often give telltale signs of inappropriate tensions: the brow will show signs of furrowing or frowning; the eyebrows twitch or lift suddenly as the singer approaches certain pitches; the expression of the eyes will show apprehension, fright, or even terror. These tensions, in addition to revealing the singer's state of mind, also often accompany postural faults of the neck and upper back.

The lips can form exaggerated shapes and will sometimes be seen to quiver. They will seem to be harshly or aggressively set so the face adopts a fixed and often dramatically inappropriate expression. They can also be pulled strongly away from the teeth in a 'snarl' or held very firmly over the teeth. These actions, which can be the product of some exaggerated concept of resonance or articulation, also seem to be a byproduct of neck and jaw misuse.

Tongue

Commonly, the tongue can be seen to be retracting, by bunching up and withdrawing the tip away from the lower teeth, or with the tip tilting up towards the roof of the mouth. This latter action is often observed on the higher notes. In more extreme cases, the tongue may withdraw into the mouth so that it is never visible, even on the most open vowels.

Larynx and jaw

The larynx position can be a sign of vocal strain if it appears to be forced down when the chin is depressed or pulled up when the jaw is thrust forward. Some singers use an exaggerated depression of the larynx to produce a darker, more dramatic tonal quality.

The musculature beneath the chin (the suprahyoid muscles) may be hypertonic in association with inappropriate larynx and jaw positions.

Breathing action

Breathing patterns provide auditory and visual cues to vocal disorders. Noisy inhalation with a change in body balance and weight distribution will indicate an accumulation of tensions from the previous vocal phrase and often point to technical problems much more far-reaching than just the act of breathing. Inhalation accompanied by sudden changes in facial expression could herald similar problems especially with respect to head, neck, and jaw usage. Inhalation accompanied by a sudden upward jerk of the head or raising of the shoulders may indicate breathing patterns that are focused too high in the torso and do not emphasize the essential lower rib–upper abdominal action.

9.1.2 Sound

The differing styles of classical, musical theatre, and 'pop' music, require that the singer produce a wide range of tonal qualities. For classical singers there is a demand to maximize the resonance of the voice and find a mode of production that will allow them to find an accommodation between resonance and clear diction over a wide working range of pitches.

For musical theatre singers the major demand appears to be related to direct communication of the text and, in this style, tonal quality will always take second place to diction and the word.

In the 'pop' field, the sound demand can range all the way from coarse and frantic, to mellow, laid back, and sentimental. In this range of demands the diction can go from completely unintelligible to crystal clear. The world of pop music covers a wide range of performance styles and within this diverse field one can encounter performers whose skill levels range from the advanced to the untutored and technically inept.

Although a wide variety of tonal and articulatory demands are reflected in the different vocal genres, some general guidelines can be given for indentifying poor vocal production based on the vocal sound.

Diction

The words are distorted and unclear in mid-range singing; vowel shapes are very different from those used in speech; some vowels appear to be very bright and abrasive, others dark and indistinct; the same vowel is pronounced differently within the same phrase or sequence of phrases; the words are sung with very little or no movement of the jaw and lips; the words are sung with very exaggerated, unnatural movements of the lips and jaw.

Tone quality

The tone is breathy and lacks clarity; some vowels are breathier than others; the tone is very different in quality from the top to the bottom of a one-octave scale; the resonance of the voice sounds hollow or 'booming'; the resonance of the voice sounds forced and constricted; the voice is harsh and strident, rather than vibrant and warm.

Range

The high notes seem resonant only when they are very loud; range is limited; the 'chest voice' register is forced high and sounds coarse and ugly; the man's voice cannot find any falsetto register; the woman's voice only functions in 'chest' register; sound production is guttural or breathy.

Pitch

The pitch becomes sharp with increased or decreased volume; pitch flattens with increased or decreased volume; lower notes are sharp, higher notes flat (in the female voice the reverse of this can often be the case).

Vibrato

The tone is shrill and very 'straight'; the voice has a fast nervous-sounding flutter (**tremolo**); the voice wavers over a wide space in a slow, exaggerated vibrato; the head shakes with the vibrato; the chest or abdomen shakes in time to the vibrato; vibrato appears only at the end of the note. A young singer will often use a breathy and straight tone at first. This is a symptom of inexperience and lack of coordination rather than a vocal problem.

Summary of audible errors in vocal production

- Although ugliness of tone is a subjective judgement and often related to the style of singing, many singers with serious errors in vocal production do make an ugly sound.
- Good singing should never betray great strain. Much romantic opera involves very demanding singing, but the object of technique is to make it appear controlled and easy rather than strained, shouted, or squeezed out under great pressure. Certainly there should be no evidence of great tension and strain in basic middle range scales and exercises.
- The resonance of the voice should be consistent throughout the range, in spite of the necessary shift in tonal quality that a voice must experience as it travels from the bottom to the top of its range.
- The singer should have no difficulty singing quietly and should not have to sing with great exertion to produce a loud tone.

- The words should always be clear in a comfortable mid-range.
- The vibrato should sound natural and appropriate to the volume, range, and style of the singing.

9.2 TECHNIQUES FOR REDUCING MISUSE

9.2.1 Guidelines for the Re-education of Muscle Behavior

Before considering any remedies for specific vocal faults, it is important to examine the nature of muscle behavior and the problems that attend efforts to reprogram existing patterns of usage. Many of our fundamental behavior patterns such as posture, breathing, speech, locomotion, etc. have evolved in response to either biological or social expediency in a manner that is adequate to fulfill the needs of survival and social intercourse. Obviously natural endowment and the nature of the specific task has a major bearing upon the evolving behavior pattern. The adequacy, as opposed to the efficiency, of the pattern would appear to be the overriding criterion. Hence what evolves in behaviors such as speech, posture, locomotion, etc., are actions that are idiosyncratic and to which qualitative criteria are rarely applied. In other words, as long as we can keep alive, stand up, walk around, and communicate with others, we don't ask too many questions. Our knowledge of how we achieve these things is often close to zero, and our sensory awareness of what is actually taking place is fairly limited. All this is not such an unreasonable state of affairs, for unless there is a physical breakdown of some sort, the old adage, 'If it isn't broken, don't fix it', allows people to get on with their lives without the ongoing worry of 'How am I doing this?'.

For some activities however, and singing is one of them, it is necessary to upgrade some of our patterns of action to a level of excellence, to enable the body to respond to the demands that the new activity places upon it. Athletes, dancers, and many instrumentalists are confronted with the same challenge.

In order to confront these existing patterns of usage it is necessary for us to develop a clear understanding of what constitutes good physical use and be able to compare that against the existing patterns. This can only be achieved if we can find a way to physically experience and, if possible, understand the new, desirable pattern. Only then can we be in a position to replicate a behavior with sufficient frequency to help establish a new and secure pattern of usage.

One of the situations faced by the singer in a voice-training context is that it is relatively useless to be told what not to do unless such an edict is accompanied by very clear directives about what should be done. Such directives as: 'Don't force'; 'Don't tighten your neck'; 'Don't breath so high'; 'Don't let your posture sag'; 'You don't support enough'; etc., although no doubt well meant, often do not lead to successful changes in activity as they only address what is not to be done and give no clear indications of what precisely should be happening. Only when singers can make their own comparisons between one form of usage and another can a successful basis for change be established. The task of the voice trainer therefore is to lead the singer to the experience of efficient and desirable usage of the vocal instrument. Herein lies the skill and the art of a good voice teacher, and also unfortunately the grounds for much pedagogical dispute. For example, there is a considerable body of thought that suggests that it is not a good training strategy to make the singer aware of the activity of specific muscle groups during the act of singing. The argument is based on the belief that this strategy will cause the singer to tense the particular group more than it is already. The opposite side of this debate asks how can singers change the behavior of a muscle group if they have no idea what it is doing in the first place?

In the pedagogy of the former philosophy one finds many techniques that are used to distract the singer away from the physical actions of singing. The hope is that, when distracted, singers will release some of the inhibitory behaviors that are causing inappropriate muscle use. The opposing philosophy may result in use of a more direct approach: giving specific directions as to what to do with the breathing apparatus, the tongue, the laryngeal position, the vowel form, the posture, etc.

If one can examine this situation objectively there appears to be a point where both these approaches arrive at the same place. Regardless of whether singers have traveled the distraction or the specific direction route, there is a need, when they arrive at a correct usage, to establish a clear sensory awareness of the new set of behaviors that has been established. This is what singers must be able to replicate each time they sing. If it can be reinforced by an intellectual understanding of what is going on, so much the better, but this will always remain a matter of individual choice.

It must be added, as a heartfelt opinion, that if any singers wish to go on to be teachers at some time in their careers then the intellectual understanding of precisely what is going on is not just a good idea but an absolute necessity.

Once one becomes aware that there are necessary meeting points in vocal pedagogies, then many of the pedagogic disputes will be recognized as either differences in style or in the route taken towards the same goal. Students' first and perhaps most important task is to choose the style and the route that is most compatible with their needs and personality. In this text we have chosen to offer suggestions that hail from both sides of the pedagogical argument.

9.2.2 General Suggestions for Reducing Misuse

Once singers have made their choice of teacher it is clear that they are committed to many years of study to develop and refine their technique. There are probably as many methods and strategies for teaching singing as there are teachers and there are certainly many books which detail these. It is doubtful that any but the most central and generalized issues can be dealt with in print without the intervention of the ears and experience of a good teacher. The following are some basic suggestions for helping singers to sing in a healthy and happy manner and to change any harmful habits which may have developed, followed by some more specific strategies for particular problems.

Choose a suitable repertoire

Singers with obvious vocal problems should avoid a repertoire which is very demanding in volume, tessitura and emotional intensity until they have solved the major problems. If a singer demonstrates vocal misuse on a simple, mid-range song, these will likely be compounded while negotiating an enormous vocal challenge. In fact the problems often develop as a result of repeated attempts to perform repertoire beyond a singer's ability. The natural sense of haste to succeed which ambition and enthusiasm engender must be redirected, and the wise teacher will have a very clear outline of a progression of repertoire that will lead the singer surely and carefully along the road of development.

Practice speaking well

Most singers with patterns of abuse in their singing demonstrate the same patterns in their speech. If singers cannot present a phrase easily in speech with clear, unforced diction, sustained breath, no vocal fry, good variation in inflection, appropriate pitch range, and a pleasing, even resonance, it is unlikely that they will be able to produce good results when they come to the act of singing, with its added demands of sustained pitch and rhythm. Once some of the ideal conditions are met in speaking phrases, the singer should try to speak the phrases in the rhythm of the song, but on a monotone, then add pitch. This practice has the artistic advantage of forcing the singer to consider the meaning and quality of the words when divorced from the composer's intentions. This often produces not only a greater understanding of the meaning of the text, but also a greater appreciation of the composer's achievement.

This procedure is especially important in the preparation of texts to be sung in a foreign language. A precise understanding of the articulatory requirements of the language in question is essential prior to imposing the demands of pitch, singing tone, and emotional meaning.

Practice while performing some other activity

Practicing singing while walking, bicycling, or reading may seen a rather surprising suggestion but is aimed at reducing some of the artificial, convoluted, tense habits that singers with vocal problems have developed. If singers can recognize that it is their imposed, misdirected manner of use that interferes with the natural freedom of their actions then they may be able to return to a more simple, unforced approach which can later become more sophisticated. Many problems stem from the singers' desire to produce a big, exciting tone which they have heard on records, but they have guessed wrongly about how that sound is made.

As was discussed earlier, the imagery and tonal models employed by the singer are crucial to the production of a free, resonant, vocal tone, and it is of the greatest importance that models and images are appropriate to the natural endowments and potentialities of the individual singer.

Curtail public performances

Singers with vocal problems should not continue to perform in public until the problems are solved. Even the best singers sometimes resort to desperate measures in performance because they feel pressured, and that they have no alternatives. Often the accommodations that the singer makes under these circumstances stay with the singer long after the particular causitive occasion has passed.

Learn in silence

The learning of new material can be very fatiguing on the vocal instrument. Regardless of how good a sight-reader a singer may be, this activity will always prove to be much more tiring than singing well-known and practiced repertoires. What must be remembered is that for balanced and controlled singing there needs to be precise, mental directives from brain to muscle regarding the required action. While material is being learned many of these directives are unclear. The uncertainty and anxiety which goes with that leaves the vocal instrument in anything but the optimal condition for good use. Most singers learn new material by 'throwing their voices at it' and repeatedly singing the piece, often loudly, until they feel that they have mastered it. The truth is that many of the aspects of a vocal composition can be learned with little or no sound being produced. The resolution of language pronunciation and meaning can be accomplished first in silence and then at a spoken level. Rhythmic patterns can be mastered in the same way. An understanding of the harmonic structure can be achieved in silence with the assistance of a keyboard. Even melodic patterns can be learned silently at the keyboard.

With this knowledge it is then possible for the singer to consider the breath requirements of musical phrasing and tackle the various technical requirements that a piece imposes. Only after all this has been done should singers begin to practice the piece using full voice. This will then build up the strength and stamina of the voice to enable it sustain the specific demands of that particular composition. Each new work contains its own unique structure and challenges and requires this kind of systematic approach to learning. Although not all the stress and fatigue can be removed from learning new material, a thoughtful, systematic process that reduces the amount of singing time can go a long way to minimize wear and tear.

Exercise caution over total voice use

The total amount of voice-use time and the environment wherein it is used have a major bearing upon vocal health. Even the best-used voices will experience fatigue after a period of demanding usage. At this point rest is called for. The environment of the vocal activity will contribute in a significant way to the rate of fatigue experienced, especially if the ambient noise level is high and the air quality is poor or lacking in humidity, or both. For singers this can mean loud orchestras or bands; smokey, noisy performance venues; a performance style that requires switching back and forth from speech to song; talking at parties, on airplanes; cheering at sports events; singing too loudly in a choir; trying to keep up with colleagues with larger voices.

The singer must remember that it is the summation of singing and speaking time that constitutes total voice-usage time and reasonable caution must be taken regarding both these activities.

9.2.3 Distracting, Disabling and Rebuilding

Most experienced singers with vocal problems will have built up a complex interdependent and rigid system of singing and it is sometimes very difficult to work with one part of the system at a time. Sometimes it is necessary to disable the whole system and return the singer to a child-like state not associated with singing. Simple acts such as laughing, 'agreeing' (*hmm!*, *hmm!*), humming while sitting on the floor cradling the knees, singing a nursery rhyme in a child-like voice to a child, singing a light popular song while crouching on the floor with arms wrapped around the legs, may be employed to encourage the singer to break learned patterns of poor coordination. The movement activities suggested in Chapter 11, section 11.3 could also be used in this context.

In **rebuilding** it is important to ensure that the models the singer has in mind are appropriate. Many vocal problems arise from attempts to copy other singers who have different physiques and ages. Teachers' voices are different from their students' and may have their own problems, but unfortunately frequently become the model to be emulated. Attempts to produce powerful, 'focused' tones often result in stridency and tension; attempts to produce rich, resonant tones often result in swallowed, muffled sounds. The model to be followed must provide the singer with a clear concept of physical poise, and tonal and dynamic goals that are appropriate to the natural endowments of the singer in question. To strive for anything other than the specifically appropriate will always lead to excess, and stressful demands being made upon the vocal instrument.

9.2.4 Speech Habits

The necessity for good speech habits for the singer has been stressed. Although there are differences in the purposes and physical demands of speech and singing, the transference from speech to song is of great importance, since singers with vocal problems often carry-over from speech to singing the distortion of both vowels and consonants. Often a natural coordination is encouraged by employing the good speech model in singing. This may feel wrong at first, nevertheless is a useful method of disabling the system.

9.3 INTERACTION WITH LARYNGOLOGISTS AND SPEECH PATHOLOGISTS

For many generations, singing teachers have operated in isolation, not only from other voice professionals, such as laryngologists and speech pathologists, but also from other instrumental teachers because of the very personal and hidden nature of the instrument. Svengali, in George Du Maurier's novel, *Trilby*, exerts an hypnotic hold over Trilby who, without his influence, cannot sing at all. It seems that vocal technique has, by tradition, been mysterious and extremely subjective. Great teachers produce other great teachers and the secrets are passed down through the generations. Interaction with medical professionals necessitates that singing teachers expose and examine their technical formats, in the best interests of the voice-disordered singer.

Unquestionably the most valuable interdisciplinary relationship to emerge in recent times is the interaction of the singer and voice teacher with the speech pathologist, the laryngologist, and when possible and necessary, the psychiatrist. The realization and continued confirmation that the vocal instrument is common to speech and song, and that faults in one are almost always mirrored in the other provides a perspective which discourages extremism and factionalism in pedagogy. The scientific caution and method of health professionals, whose continued confirmation that the body and mind operate as a whole and that the voice is a reflection of the whole person, bring to the singing teacher a necessary and valuable balance. The teacher becomes much more wary of making quasi-scientific justifications of methods to students and is challenged to find language from the world of singing and music to carry on discourse with the other professionals. The training of the ear and eye as diagnostic tools becomes easier in the presence of other eyes and ears with different training.

9.4 SOME FINAL THOUGHTS

The power of the interdisciplinary approach to voice care extends far-reaching benefits to singers. All aspects of singers' physical and technical processes can be evaluated including an understanding of the impact of the stresses and strains that attend the life and work of the vocal performer. A team approach ensures that all key factors are considered in the development of a rehabilitation program.

It is critical that the singer brings to such a process an openmindedness and a willingness to follow the prescribed strategy. This is not always the case and there are a number of reasons why a singer may be reluctant to consult the medical fraternity about a voice problem. He or she may be confronting a strange mixture of fear and hope upon approaching the voice-clinic team. The fear is of the unknown and what terrible tidings may await regarding the state of the vocal apparatus, which for many means the vocal folds. For many singers, nodules are often the worst possible diagnosis that can be pronounced (even cancer pales alongside these). The hope is carried that there will be some simple and quick, sometimes 'by tonight', cure. There is always word circulating in the profession of sprays and potions that will provide a quick fix for the problem and get a singer through the coming show. Although the potency of modern drugs can create the occasional minor miracle, many problems need a more far-reaching remedy than can be found in the spray or the pill. The problem that is being considered is often the product of long-term physical behavior, sometimes under adverse conditions and environments. The proposed rehabilitation strategy may well require a major re-evaluation and possible overhaul of vocal techniques, which could mean a recommended change in vocal advisers or voice teachers, or both. A change in performance conditions, frequency, and possibly even style may be necessary. For many singers such recommendations could constitute a major upheaval, and the reluctance to cooperate is understandable. The singer must confront the truth: sometimes we run out of options and there is only one sensible route despite the immediate personal and economic implications. Contrary to our fears, the periodic re-evaluation of technique and art can often lead to better and maybe greater things.

10

Anatomy and physiology of voice production

Voice production for speech is part of a psychomotor act that is the result of complex interactions among psychological and anatomical systems (Figure 10.1).

A comprehensive review of the anatomical structures involved in voice production should include those of the neuromuscular, respiratory, phonatory, resonance, and articulatory systems, including those central and peripheral neurological subsystems that initiate and coordinate the voluntary movements of speech. A detailed presentation of the structural aspects of all these system components is beyond the scope of this text. The reader is encouraged to refer to appropriate anatomical atlases to supplement the material offered in this chapter. Only aspects of normal structure and function that provide information fundamental to the nature and management of voice disorders will be presented in detail.

10.1 FUNCTION OF PHONATION IN VERBAL COMMUNICATION

Phonation is a term used to refer to the production of sound waves by vibration of structures within the larynx: under normal circumstances the true vocal folds are the primary vibrators. Phonation with the true vocal folds is also referred to as the 'glottic source' of a speech sound, the 'glottis' being the space between the vocal folds, on the same horizontal plane. Phonation provides the quasi-regular sound component that gives speech audible or musical tone. The vowel and vowel-like phonemes (linguistic sound 'segments') of English are always characterized by phonation, and are the loudest, most intense components in the speech signal. The phonatory system also provides mechanisms for 'devoicing' phonemes that are not associated with vocal tone (and so require that the vocal folds are not vibrating during their production), primarily by contraction of the posterior crico-arytenoid muscles, the intrinsic vocal fold abductors (the muscles that pull the vocal folds apart). The devoicing mechanism is most active for the voiceless phonemes such as the English /p/, /f/, /θ/, /t/, /s/, /tʃ/, /ʃ/, and /k/.

In addition to providing tone for voiced speech sounds, phonation for speech

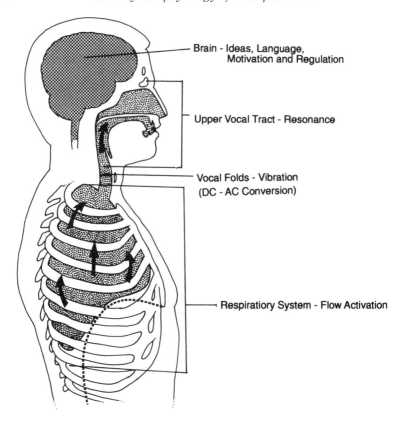

Figure 10.1 Mechanisms involved in voice production for speech.

includes pitch and loudness mechanisms that create intonation and stress (known as **suprasegmental** features of speech) to help listeners determine the meaning and emotional intent of speech. The suprasegmental function of voice is diverse and fascinating! By continuously adjusting laryngeal factors such as vocal fold length and tension, and other parameters such as vocal tract length, and the rate and amount of airflow from the lungs, we can produce innumerable combinations of vocal frequencies, intensities, and qualities during speech. We can change the semantics (meaning) and syntax (grammar) of a sentence, just by altering the pitch inflections, or patterns of emphasis. These speech attributes are largely based on phonatory function. In addition, we can readily alter the mood and intent of a communicative utterance by varying loudness, pitch, and quality of the voice, without making a single change to the words.

The biological systems for respiration, phonation, resonance, and articulation work together in complex ways during speech. It is therefore difficult to provide accurate and comprehensive descriptions of single component functions of this complex psychomotor act. It is helpful, however, to consider certain aspects of individual system components for the purposes of evaluation and treatment of voice disorders.

10.2 NEUROMUSCULAR SYSTEMS INVOLVED IN SPEECH AND PHONATION

The true organ of speech and voice is the brain, and to try and describe all the systems involved would be presumptuous. But it may be helpful in understanding voice disorders for us to trace some of the paths that a thought may take from its inception to its expression.

First, a thought consists of both intellectual and emotional elements that, when coupled to the underlying personality and style of the speaker, set up the postural and muscle tonus patterns required to deliver the utterance with the needed features. The clinician who is presented with the task of evaluating a voice-disordered patient must keep this thought/feeling/speech interface in mind, since it is here that the source of disorders frequently lies, and this fact may get lost in the myriad of voice and speech science detail described herein. Chapter 5 covers the area in more detail.

Secondly, humans use a neuromuscular system for voice generation that initially evolved for other purposes including swallowing, breathing, and airway control. The clinician needs to bear in mind that the larynx, pharynx, and esophagus form an embryologically related neuromuscular tube that is controlled partly voluntarily and partly involuntarily. Sensorimotor reflexes from the pharynx, larynx and esophagus to the brain, and back again, are clearly very important, to the extent that voice clinicians tend to form strong reductive biases about the influence of medical factors on voice, such as the effects of chronic gastro-esophageal reflux.

Thirdly, the neuromuscular activities needed to produce a voice must be delicately coordinated. The vocal athletic gift has been more heavily bestowed on some than others, as has the ability to hit a baseball or dance. But training in these skills can enhance voice production of the voice user who has less natural talent, as well as the gifted one, and much of this book is dedicated to this end.

Structures of the central and peripheral nervous system are responsible for the act of speech. Within the cerebral cortex, the areas generally recognized as being important to speech and language processing and formulation are the left inferior frontal gyrus of the frontal lobe (**Broca's area**); the left angular gyrus of the parietal lobe, and the left superior temporal gyrus, and the temporo parietal region (**Wernicke's area**). These areas receive input from other cortical and subcortical processing areas as well, including structures of the limbic system (the emotional center), while one is engaging in verbal discourse. Within the cerebral cortex, the precentral gyrus is also of great importance to verbal communication, since it houses the cell bodies of the motor nerves that operate skeletal muscles during voluntary movements such as speech. The postcentral gyrus is an area for processing various types of sensory input, for example, proprioceptive information regarding the state of muscles and direction and degree of movements. Within the basal ganglia of the subcortex are important motor and sensory relay and coordination areas such as in the thalamus. The cerebellum also plays a role in achieving finely tuned coordinated movements.

Most of the peripheral cranial nerves play a part in speech and voice production. Any disease process that results in paralysis of cranial nerves, in any combination, will have significant effects on speech and voice.

The **fifth**, or trigeminal nerve, has a major motor component in its mandibular division, which supplies the muscles of mastication, and those in the anterior floor of the mouth. We have shown in Chapter 1, section F.2, detailed evidence as to how jaw and suprahyoid muscle tension are a factor in voice misuse.

The **seventh**, or facial nerve, supplies the facial muscles of expression which are obviously a big part of verbal and nonverbal communication. The lips, served by this nerve, are important speech articulators.

The **eighth**, or hearing nerve, plays an important sensory role in monitoring speech and is the afferent (sensory input) component of many sensorimotor reflex arcs.

The **ninth**, or glossopharyngeal nerve, supplies sensation to much of the posterior oral cavity and to the pharynx, as well as the motor supply to some palatal and pharyngeal muscles. Thus it plays an important role in resonance.

The **tenth**, or vagus nerve, is 'king' of the throat, serving both sensory and motor functions to the entire pharyngolaryngo-esophageal tube. The superior laryngeal branch of the vagus nerve provides sensation to the larynx and pharynx, as well as motor function to the paired crico-thyroid muscles, the muscles of 'vocal pitch'. The remainder of the intrinsic laryngeal muscles receive their motor innervation from the recurrent laryngeal nerve, also a branch of the vagus nerve. In addition to innervating the intrinsic laryngeal muscles, the vagus supplies the autonomic function to minor salivary glands, gastric acid secretors, and to plexi (nerve networks) that control peristalsis (swallowing movements).

The **eleventh**, or accessory nerve, gives motor supply to the trapezius and sternocleidomastoid muscles. We have seen how the trapezius and short rotators of the neck are overactive in several patterns of voice misuse.

Finally the **twelfth**, or hypoglossal nerve, sends motor input to the tongue, the most complex speech articulator. It also combines with some fibers of the cervical plexus to supply the strap muscles of the neck.

The cervical and phrenic plexi (nerve bundles) of the peripheral spinal nerve system need also to be considered for their importance in supporting muscles of respiration and speech-breathing.

An important component to voice function is the role of servomechanisms or feedback devices within the structures of respiration, phonation, resonance, and articulation. These may be in the form of fine hair cells (**cilia**) within the respiratory system that are sensitive to air pressure changes, or muscle spindles within the main muscles that detect the state of contraction of the main muscle, and may also be sensitive to tactile, vibratory, and aerodynamic changes in the vocal tract.

It is imperative that the voice clinician, from whichever parent discipline, maintains a good working understanding of the neuro-anatomical connections of the upper aerodigestive tract, and particularly of those portions that serve speech and voice. The reader is referred to the many excellent anatomical texts and atlases listed at the end of this chapter, for further details.

10.3 FUNCTIONS OF THE RESPIRATORY SYSTEM: 'SPEECH-BREATHING'

10.3.1 Nature of the Mechanism: an Overview

The process of phonation engages the basic structures of the upper and lower respiratory systems. Voice for speech and singing is produced principally during the exhalation phase of respiration.

Readers who are unfamiliar with terms related to respiration are referred to the glossary in section 10.3.4.

In its simplest conceptualization, speech-breathing functions to maintain a relatively constant flow of air to overcome resistance offered by the closed glottis (the area between the vocal folds) and thus to provide the aerodynamic driving force throughout phonation. In addition, the expiratory flow must provide appropriate aerodynamic forces to allow for the oral, pharyngeal, and laryngeal articulatory effects such as **plosive-aspirate** and **fricative** noises: plosive-aspirate sounds are associated with sudden release of air by an articulator, as when the lips are parted (p^h); fricative noise is the hissing sound that is created when air rushes between two articulators that are closely approximated, say the upper teeth and the lower lip, and creates air turbulence (*ffff*).

The tissues of the lungs and the rib-cage structures have inherent elastic properties that allow them to be stretched, and provide recoil forces making them want to return to their respective 'rest' positions after they are stretched. While the tissues are being stretched, they are storing passive energy that is used in the recoil forces. For example, the lungs have a passive recoil force that makes them want to shrink in volume after they are stretched for inhalation (the in-breath). The rib-cage structure, on the other hand, has a recoil force that makes it tend to expand back to its neutral rest position after it is pulled in during exhalation (the out-breath), or to reduce its dimensions if it is expanded beyond its rest position during inhalation. These recoil forces are capitalized on to a large degree during quiet respiration (non speech tidal breathing), and vary as a function of lung volume. The respiratory system also engages voluntary muscles to enhance inhalation and exhalation activities. Both passive elastic recoil forces, and active muscular forces are involved in the maintenance of appropriate expiratory airflow and subglottic air pressures required for phonation to occur. Subglottic pressures (pressures below the glottis) are determined by airflow rate and laryngeal, or supralaryngeal resistance (resistance in structures above the glottis). During conversational speech at normal loudness, subglottic pressures of from 5–12 cm H_2O are required to maintain phonation.

Figure 10.3 provides a prototype relaxation curve demonstrating directions and degrees of overall relaxation pressures or forces (P_r) throughout the vital capacity. At resting expiratory level (REL) P_r is 0; above REL, P_r is positive; and below REL, P_r is

The Speech Breathing Mechanism

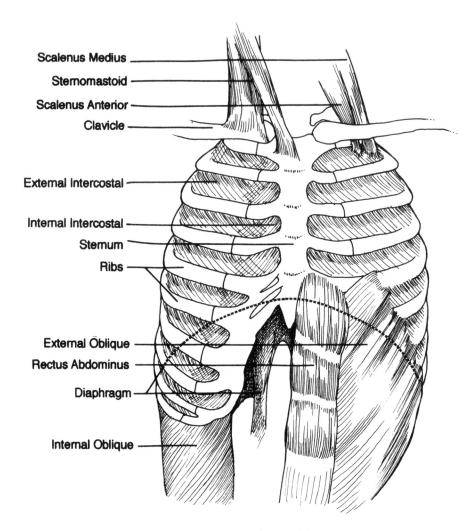

Figure 10.2 Primary structures for speech-breathing.

negative. The relationship of a relaxation curve to force components of the chest wall for various loudness dynamics is shown in Figure 11.5.

Figure 10.4 estimates the degree to which passive or relaxation-recoil forces in the respiratory system are available to provide the necessary subglottic pressure for speech over time, within the typical vital capacity range employed for conversation, typically from 60% to 30% of total lung volume. Clearly, a constant subglottic pressure of 7 cm

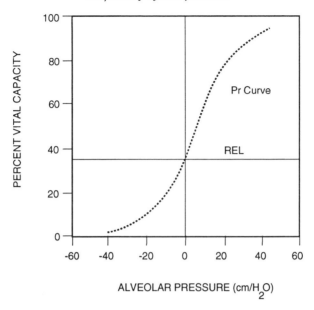

Figure 10.3 A prototype relaxation curve (see text for detailed description). (After Weismer [62], with permission.)

H_2O could be maintained for only a small part of the vital capacity should one rely only on passive forces of the respiratory system. As we will see in the next section, use of the passive expiratory forces during speech-breathing is not simple, nor are interactions between use of passive and active respiratory forces.

Any internal or external situations that require changes in loudness, pitch, or voice quality affect subglottic pressure demands; for example, loud or emotive speech is generally produced with higher subglottic pressure.

In reality, the speech-breathing mechanism must perform a much more complicated task than simply supplying a relatively constant flow of air to maintain steady phonation. Within a spoken phrase, the segmental (single sound unit) and suprasegmental demands of verbal communication result in constantly changing aerodynamic 'loading' forces. The segmental characteristics of speech require continual changes in articulatory shapes, which in turn affect intraoral pressures and flows and ultimately result in recognizable sound sequences, or speech phrases. Articulatory adjustments resulting in 'speech' cause fluctuations in supraglottic loading pressures, which in turn change resistances at the glottis and may even affect vocal fold vibratory patterns. The most dramatic examples of articulatory maneuvers that offer rapid resistance changes within the supraglottic vocal tract during speech, are the plosive sounds such as /p/ or /t/, and fricative sounds such as /s/ or /f/. Since subglottic pressure should remain relatively constant for phonation to have consistent loudness, pitch, and quality, the aerodynamic driving forces of the respiratory mechanism must

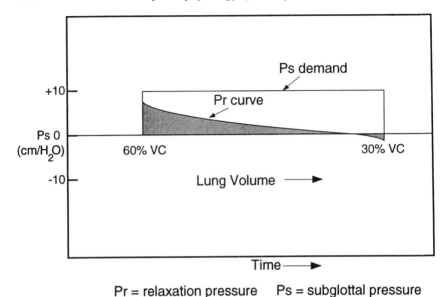

Pr = relaxation pressure   Ps = subglottal pressure

Figure 10.4 Availability of relaxation pressures in the respiratory system to meet subglottic pressure requirements for speech over time and lung volume (see text for detailed description). P_r = relaxation presure; P_s = subglottic pressure. (After Weismer [62], with permission.)

have ways of compensating for the changes in vocal tract loading forces, to stabilize phonatory function. On the other hand, suprasegmental effects of intonation (inflection), or stress (emphasis) require that the respiratory system can adjust quickly to contribute to altered subglottic pressure demands and make these changes possible.

Since subglottic pressure during phonation is determined by both respiratory forces and laryngeal resistance, adjustments must be made to the respiratory forces to compensate for, or overcome glottic resistance in cases where valving at the glottis is compromised or exaggerated. Conversely, if respiratory forces are somehow compromised or exaggerated, the muscles influencing glottic closure may attempt to compensate for or balance the driving forces in order to maintain phonation.

Our current understanding of mechanics of the respiratory system for speech production embraces the concept of **motor equivalence**. That is to say, a wide variance in mechanical patterns within the breathing system is observed across individuals when they prepare for, initiate and sustain phonation during speech [17]. Furthermore, patterns of breathing for singing and theatrical voice use may differ significantly from those associated with speech-breathing [17, 18, 20, 59, 60]. Individual variation in patterns may be explained by factors such as body type, training, and vocal performance style. Given the many influences on motor equivalence contributing to differences in speech-breathing style, we must question the validity of voice training and therapy techniques that use the exact speech-breathing style of the teacher or therapist as the primary model for all students or patients.

10.3.2 Respiratory Kinematics and Dynamics

Traditionally, speech physiologists have differentiated between two functional parts of the respiratory system to study speech-breathing: the rib cage and the diaphragm-abdomen. Together, these two functional units comprise the 'chest wall'. This delineation continues to be useful in understanding speech-breathing.

Modern concepts of speech-breathing are based largely on the techniques of **kinematics** (movement patterns) and **dynamics** (muscular-force functions), first developed by Hixon and collaborators [18, 19] in the early 1970s for application to speech research. Both techniques use a relaxation curve as a reference for each individual's speech-breathing function. Voluntary closure of the glottis along with relaxation of all respiratory muscles allows for static measures to be made for each individual's reference curves. In the case of kinematic measures, the relaxation curve represents relative positions of displacement for the abdomen and rib cage at various lung volumes. For the dynamic measures, the relaxation curve represents relative pressures within the abdominal and rib-cage cavities of the chest wall at various lung volumes.

The relaxation reference charts are assumed to be relatively constant for an individual, although body orientation, such as upright versus supine (lying on the back) position, will affect the shape of the curve significantly due to differing gravitational effects on the abdomen and rib cage. In addition, both developmental and aging factors will have an impact on the elasticity and capacity of the involved tissues. Taken together, the relaxation curves describe the non muscular passive chest wall displacement force potentials associated with two recoil reactions over a time–volume history, for a specified body orientation. The two relaxation functions include the natural elastic tendency of the lung tissue to compress the air inside the lungs, creating a positive, 'pleural' pressure, and the opposing tendency of the chest wall structures to expand creating a negative pressure in the lungs. Together with the effects of gravity and abdominal hydraulics, these forces create a passive, 'summation' force. In order to serve as an accurate reference for muscular contributions of speech-breathing, it is important that relaxation summation functions be plotted throughout the relevant ranges of vital capacity for a given posture since the degree of displacement or force varies with lung volume as well as posture (e.g. standing versus lying supine).

For the kinematic measures, magnetometers or strain gauges can be used to measure relative movements of the rib cage and the abdominal wall and thus used to estimate volume displacements in the lungs (Figure 10.5). Measures, in voltages, of changes in chest-wall displacements for the rib cage and abdomen during speech can be plotted on an x–y graph, which uses as a reference, the relaxation curve for the speaker in the same posture (Figure 10.6). Any deviations from the relaxation curve are considered representative of active muscular dynamics, and the direction of the deviation implies which part of the chest wall was moving or providing force (Figure 10.6).

Dynamic measures are generally made with pressure transducers measuring pressures from catheter balloons placed below and above the diaphragm, one in the stomach and one in the esophagus. Since this procedure is invasive, less data is available

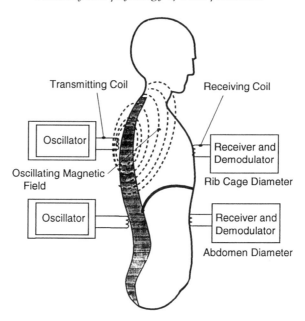

Figure 10.5 Hardware design for measuring kinematics of the chest wall with magnetometers. (After Baken) [4], with permission.

for study than for kinematic measures. Results of pressure deviations can be plotted in a manner similar to the motion–motion diagrams for each individual, for a variety of speech and phonation tasks. The plots provide information regarding the amount and direction of muscular force. Hixon and colleagues have demonstrated that kinematic measures can be used to estimate active forces of individual chest wall parts during speech-breathing. For detailed descriptions of measurement techniques and interpretations the reader is directed to texts by Baken [4] and Hixon [17].

Taken together, these sets of speech-breathing measures can provide valuable information about patterns of movement and aerodynamics from which we infer roles of the various structures and muscles of the respiratory system. Figure 10.7 summarizes the relevant pressures, volume displacements and movements to be considered in describing speech-breathing.

In addition to measures of volume displacements and pressures within the chest wall, a limited number of surface electromyographic (EMG) studies have been undertaken to contribute towards our understanding of breathing for speech and performance. These have included studies of activity in the intercostal and abdominal muscles, and the diaphragm [36, 37, 47, 61].

10.3.3 What Do We Know About Speech-Breathing?

The following observations have been confirmed in several studies of speech-breathing, and contribute to our current understanding of the mechanisms involved.

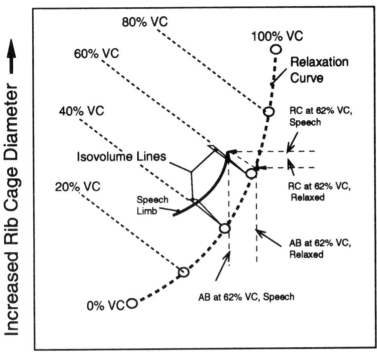

Figure 10.6 Hypothetical expiratory limb for a speech utterance from kinematic measures using magnetometers. VC = vital capacity; RC = rib cage; AB = abdomen. The relaxation reference curve is produced by filling the lungs to a specified volume then relaxing all voluntary musculature so only the passive recoil forces are influencing chest wall shape. The isovolume lines represent the range of chest wall shapes at a specified volume when contained air is shifted from the abdomen to rib cage and vice versa. Vertical shifts indicate rib cage contributions, and horizontal shifts indicate abdominal contributions. By plotting 'speech limbs' of relative contributions of the different chest wall parts we can study the individual characteristics of speech-breathing and compare patterns of speech-breathing across individuals. A sample speech limb is represented by the darkest line, extending from 62% to 30% vital capacity. In this example, muscular abdominal forces are engaged at the outset of the phrase, as demonstrated by the limb placement left of the relaxation reference curve at 62%; abdominal contributions to the speech phrase are demonstrated by leftward excursion of the limb over time and volume, and rib cage contributions are demonstrated by downward excursion of the limb. For this hypothetical speaker, it can be seen that the contribution of the rib cage displacement is large for the first part of the phrase, followed by an increase in abdominal displacement in the latter half. (After Weismer [62], with permission.)

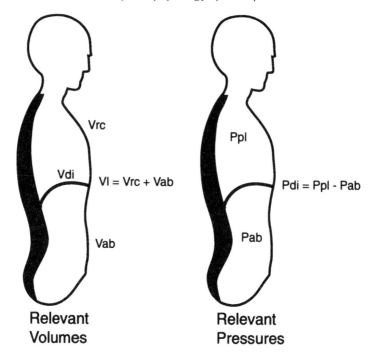

Figure 10.7 Relevant volume displacements and pressures of concern for a comprehensive analysis of chest wall function during speech. v = volume displacement; P = pressure. Subscripts for relevant volumes are: di = diaphragm; rc = rib cage wall; l = lung; ab = abdominal wall. Subscripts for relevant pressures are: pl = pleural; ab = abdominal; di = transdiaphragmatic. (After Hixon, Mead, and Goldman [19], with permission.)

Inspiration for speech

Inspiration for speech involves activity in the diaphragm and external intercostal muscles. In cases where a large inspiration is required, and often in association with voice disorders, a variety of accessory muscles may be used to facilitate rib-cage elevation. The so-called **inspiratory** muscles may be used in special ways during voice performance such as singing [34, 35].

Maintenance of subglottal pressure for speech

Both the rib cage and abdominal mechanisms contribute to maintenance of alveolar pressure (pressure within the lungs) during speech. The internal intercostal muscles are of particular importance in maintaining a fairly steady pressure to ensure constant airflow within the middle range of lung volume.

Abdominal muscle activity

The abdominal muscles are active in all individuals at the outset of phonation for speech and singing [17–22, 25, 59, 60, 62, 63]. This appears to be the case even when phonation is initiated at lung volumes where relaxation forces alone would be adequate to provide sufficient subglottic pressure under normal conversational situations. Of particular importance to voice production are activity in the internal and external oblique abdominal muscles, which pull the rib cage downward and push the abdominal wall inward on contraction; and the transverse abdominal muscle, which pushes the abdominal wall inward on contraction. Weismer [62] has provided theoretical support for the mechanical advantages of using abdominal muscle forces during speech. He has suggested that the abdominal muscle tone exerts pressure on the diaphragm, which in turn provides a counter force to rib-cage compression forces, primarily the internal intercostal muscles, to make them more effective. Without the abdominal pressure, activity of the internal intercostals would result in downward displacement of the diaphragm, and no significant expiratory driving force. This counterforce role may be particularly important for the rapid pulsatile movements during speech. The upward pressure on the diaphragm may also ensure that it returns to a neutral position following inspiration. Since voluntary muscles contract most efficiently from rest position this force facilitates rapid diaphragmatic contractions required for quick inspirations during speech.

Prephonatory posturing of the respiratory system

An expanded rib cage is often noted at onset, and throughout speech and singing, compared to the position noted for the same lung volume on a relaxation-curve. (Figure 10.6) This is represented by a higher position of the speech-limb onset compared with the vertical position for the same lung volume on the relaxation curve. This position must involve use of muscle groups generally labelled as inspiratory muscles, in particular the external intercostal muscles, although speech is thought to be an 'expiratory' activity. It appears to contradict previous theory that opposing forces, abdominal-expiratory and rib-cage-inspiratory, do not co-occur in speech-breathing [62].

Comparisons across individuals suggest that no single typical pattern exists for prephonatory posturing and speech-breathing excepting the observation that abdominal muscles are engaged at the outset of a speech phrase. Several possible combinations of individual chest wall activities have been demonstrated in prephonatory posturing [21, 63]. During speech phonation, speech limbs are almost horizontal on the graph for some individuals, suggesting that the predominant activity during the speech phrase is abdominal. Others appear to use predominantly rib-cage activity for speech after the initial abdominal and rib-cage posturing efforts. Figure 10.8 demonstrates speech-breathing movement patterns for two different individuals across three different loudness or effort levels. For the first individual, the speech limbs for several successive sentences indicate a predominance of abdominal displacement, and

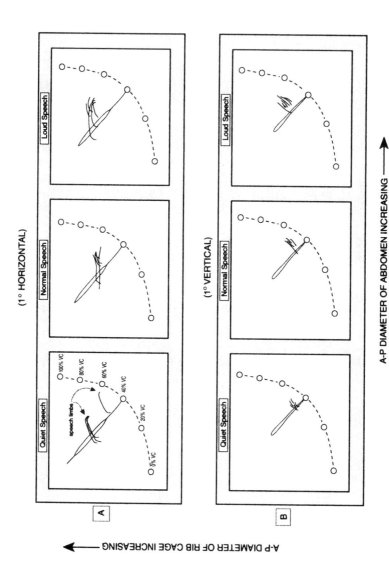

Figure 10.8 Speech limbs for two different speakers under three different speech effort levels. Speaker A demonstrates predominantly abdominal movements during speech as represented by horizontal speech limb movement. Speaker B demonstrates predominantly rib cage movements during speech as represented by vertical speech limb movement. (After Hixon [17], with permission.)

for the second individual, the speech limbs are principally vertical, indicating predominance of rib-cage movement. These movement patterns are consistent for each individual across different phonation loudness tasks.

Individual variation related to body type and aging

Recently, a great interest has developed in the influence of body type on speech-breathing, and some general trends have emerged. Lean males, or ectomorphs, tend to use more rib cage activity than abdominal, whereas for endomorphs (more rotund individuals) the opposite is true. In addition paradoxical rib-cage movements have been noted in endomorphs [23]. In some studies, women and men have been noted to have different speech-breathing patterns [22, 25, 63]; however, a survey of all studies suggests no consistent sex-based differences, the apparent differences perhaps being related more to body type.

Geriatric adults initiate speech at higher lung and rib-cage volumes, use higher lung and rib-cage excursions, and some use larger degrees of vital capacity per syllable than do younger adults [24, 25]. Apart from known physiological changes in the respiratory system, the speech-breathing changes may be partly explainable on the basis of laryngeal changes. Geriatrics, especially men, may experience difficulty approximating their vocal folds completely due to muscle atrophy, and thus may need to compensate with larger lung volumes and rib-cage excursions to meet voicing and linguistic demands.

Variability of lung volumes used in speech

During normal speech, most individuals begin a phrase at a lung volume about equal to 60% of the vital capacity, but a wide variability has been noted in the lung volume at which individuals finish speech phrases. Some go below the resting expiratory level, using some of their functional residual capacity (FRC). This individual variability may be explained in part by developmental, aging and body-type factors. Children have less muscular strength than adults, and therefore may be more likely to use FRC during speech. Geriatrics have reduced vital capacities, increased residual volumes and sometimes reduced glottic valving capabilities, thus they may tend to impinge less or more on residual volumes, depending on system flexibility or degree of laryngeal compensation for an incompetent glottis, or both. For vocal performance, much larger percentages of the vital capacity may be employed.

Variability related to phonatory task

There is evidence that the respiratory-system activities for singing, chanting, and other nonconversational 'speech' may be quite different than accounted for above [18, 20, 34, 35, 44, 47, 59, 60]. This may be due to the different duration-timing, prosody, pitch, and intensity requirements of these vocal activities, and also may be related to the different psycho-emotional motivations behind each activity. Hixon and colleagues [18, 19] have described different speech-breathing pattern demands for sustained phonation or steady speech activities compared with patterns noted for conversational speech. Activities such as recitation of serial numbers, which are non-emotional, and have limited suprasegmental demands, may use much larger ranges of lung volume and take greater advantage of relaxation characteristics or passive expiratory forces, in combination with inspiratory 'checking' forces. For vocal performance, as in singing or theatrical voice use, training is likely to have a large influence on the phonatory breathing patterns. This is discussed further in Chapter 11.

Variability related to physical and emotional changes

Respiratory function for speech is highly susceptible to changes in physical and emotional states.

Body posture and alignment factors can greatly influence speech-breathing function. For example, predictable differences in gravitational influence on respiratory function are observed in upright versus supine position [18, 48]. Sundberg and colleagues [48] demonstrated that singers used specific compensatory adjustments to adapt to changes in body position. More subtle differences in body alignment can influence rib-cage and abdominal excursion and lung volumes, and thus affect speech-breathing patterns.

The **respiratory and laryngeal systems** work together to produce sufficient subglottic pressure to meet the demands for vocal fold vibration and breath stream resistance produced by supraglottic articulators during speech. Because interaction with the phonatory system is an integral part of speech-breathing, changes to the laryngeal and supralaryngeal structures may cause compensatory changes in use of the respiratory system during speech. Overvalving or undervalving of the vocal folds during voice production will alter the subglottic pressure requirements for sustained vocal fold vibration, and therefore the force that various respiratory structures need to contribute to create the expiratory breath stream will change. Similarly, long-term changes in resistance created by articulatory or resonance structures, such as the tongue or soft palate, change the demand on the respiratory system for speech-breathing. For example, reduced articulatory dynamics or velopharyngeal incompetence will alter demands on the respiratory system during speech due to reduced supraglottic resistance during speech. In some speakers experiencing such supraglottal compromises, compensatory valving may be created within the larynx to help regulate the aerodynamic pressures. In contrast, if articulatory pressures are increased, as with stuttering, focal dystonias or muscle-misuse voice disorders, the respiratory forces must be increased to overcome high levels of glottic and supraglottic resistance.

Emotional states which result in muscular tension and altered motivation for communication can affect function of the respiratory, phonatory, and speech systems due to chronic hypertonicity of muscles normally involved in speech-breathing, phonation and articulation.

Compensatory mechanisms

Because of a degree of functional redundancy in the speech-breathing system, remarkable compensations can be observed in individuals with anatomical changes in the respiratory system, allowing it to support near-normal speech and voice function.

Servomechanisms in speech-breathing

The physiological mechanisms that are responsible for 'pulsatile' (rapidly changing) speech aerodynamic events are not fully understood, but are likely very complex, and probably involve two main types of nerve–muscle systems: extrafusal (large muscle fibers outside the muscle spindle); and intrafusal (fibers inside the muscle spindle). The extrafusal system likely includes alpha motor neuron systems of both the internal and external intercostal muscles. In cases of more emotive or emphatic speech, other muscles, for example, abdominals, may also be involved. The intrafusal muscle system may act as a servomechanism (feedback device): in this role a gamma-loop mechanism would operate in response to detection of rapid loading/unloading forces on the respiratory driving pump, and function to stabilize primary respiratory muscles during these changes, allowing for refinement of compensatory muscular adjustments. Since speech is a motor skill, it is proposed that learned patterns of interaction between the different neuromuscular systems are used to regulate the respiratory pump during the complex act of verbal communication [17].

10.3.4 Glossary for Respiration

Expiratory reserve volume (ERV)   Quantity of air that can be exhaled beyond that of tidal volume.

Functional residual capacity (FRC)   Volume of air in the respiratory system at resting expiratory level (when recoil forces of compression/expansion are at balance). In young healthy adult males, a mean FRC of 2.3 liters (2300 ml) is estimated.

Inspiratory capacity   Maximum volume that can be inhaled from the resting expiratory level.

Inspiratory reserve volume (IRV)   Quantity of air that can be inhaled beyond that in tidal volume.

Residual volume   Quantity of air that remains after a maximum exhalation.

Resting expiratory level (REL)   Volume of air in the lungs allowing for a pressure balance between the elastic recoil compression forces of the lungs and the recoil expansion forces of the thorax structure. REL also refers to the typical volume at the end of a exhalation phase of rest breathing.

Tidal volume   Quantity of air inhaled and exhaled during one cycle of respiration – generally in reference to rest breathing. The 'normal' in adults ranges from 0.5 to 0.75

liters (during sedentary activity levels), and occurs approximately 12 times a minute. This represents approximately 10% of the vital capacity.

Total lung capacity (TLC)   The volume of air in the lungs after a maximum inspiration, or at the top of inspiratory capacity.

Vital capacity (VC)   Volume of air that can be exhaled following deep inhalation (after inspiratory capacity is reached, or from total lung capacity). Normal VC for adults ranges from 3.5 liters for small females, to 5 liters for average young males.

10.4 PHONATION: CONVERSION OF DC TO AC ENERGY

Phonation, or sound-producing vocal fold vibration, is a process by which DC (direct current) aerodynamic energy is converted to AC (alternating current) acoustic energy. This takes place when the vocal folds are adducted sufficiently to offer an adequate resistance to the DC airflow, so that they are set into vibration. The vocal fold adducting muscles: principally, the lateral crico-arytenoids and interarytenoids accomplish the task of approximating the arytenoid cartilages, which effects prephonatory vocal fold closure in the posterior glottis. The degree of resistance offered by the vocal folds determines how much pressure is required from the airflow to initiate and sustain vibratory action. Remember that resistance can be altered at the larynx by varying the tension and/or the degree of adduction, including that resulting from supraglottic constrictions. This determines then, in part, how hard the respiratory forces must 'work' to help sustain phonation. Other influences over the laryngeal resistance are the intended or required loudness and pitch ranges of a speech or singing phrase, and even more subtle linguistic, emotional, and pragmatic requirements. Various combinations of intrinsic muscle contractions serve to adjust the tone, length, shape, and elasticity of the vocal folds according to pitch, loudness, and quality requirements of the phonatory act. The result of the vocal fold vibration is a series of pressure pulses which disturbs the air molecules in the vocal tract so that they oscillate (alternate compression and rarefaction of the molecules). We refer to the oscillating air column as a sound pressure wave. The shape of the vocal tract resonators determines which components of the glottic source waveform will be enhanced and which will be damped, and thus the nature of sounds we will perceive. The human hearing system is sensitive to the sound pressure changes and responds, first mechanically, then in turn by sending electrophysiological signals to the brain regarding the nature of the sound.

10.4.1 Histology and Biomechanics of the Vocal Folds

In the normally speaking adult, the paired vocal folds consist of several layers of tissues which are quite different in their histological (cellular) structures. Figure 10.9 represents the histology of an adult vocal fold schematically, as studied from a mid-membranous frontal section. The most superficial layer comprises stratified squamous epithelium bordered by pseudostratified ciliated epithelium on the superior and inferior edges. The next three layers comprise the **lamina propria**. The superficial layer, also known as Reinke's space, consists of very pliable areolar tissue, which allows the mechanical

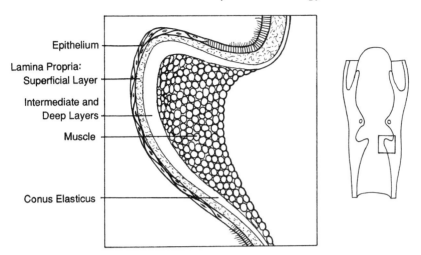

Epithelium

Lamina Propria:
Superficial Layer

Intermediate and
Deep Layers

Muscle

Conus Elasticus

Figure 10.9 Histological structure of the adult vocal fold.

'cover' to glide easily over the deeper layers of the vocal folds during vibration. The intermediate layer of the lamina propria consists predominantly of elastic tissues, and the deep layer consists mainly of collagen. The intermediate and deep layers are poorly differentiated at their borders, but the tissues are increasingly stiffer, compared to the superficial layer. Together they form the **vocal ligament**, a structure that is important during phonation for its elastic biomechanical properties. The deepest layer of the vocal fold consists of striated muscle fibers, the most viscous (stiffest) of the mechanical structures. The most medial muscle section is often referred to as the **vocalis** muscle, and the more lateral fibers comprise the **thyro-arytenoid** muscles. As is evident in Figure 10.9, the layered structure becomes simpler at the superior and inferior borders. Inferior to, and continuous with the vocal ligament, the single-layered conus elasticus provides a sheet-like support for the lower portion of the vocal fold. Neither the vocal ligament nor the conus elasticus are evident in the first few years of life.

The vocal folds are designed for efficient and effective vibration for phonatory activities. The progressive density and viscosity of the layers serves to provide a delicate and complex mechanical vibrator system. The tissue fibres for most of the layers run in anterior-to-posterior directions, or parallel to the vocal fold margins. Even the laryngeal vascular system provides design features that enhance the complex vibratory behavior: within the medial portions of the superficial layers of the vocal folds that undergo greatest excursion during phonation, the blood vessels are thinnest, and run longitudinally, thus providing uniform density, and maximum flexibility for vocal fold vibration. The tissues are stiffest in a longitudinal direction and most pliable in a transverse direction. The structure of the true vocal fold determines that the greatest flexibility for vibration is at the medial portion of the vocal folds. [12–14, 16].

The 'cover–body' theory helps explain some aspects of vocal fold vibration, by relating it to mechanical properties of the different layers and their interactions. In this theory, at least two distinct layers are described from a mechanical point of view: the 'cover' comprising the epithelium and superficial layer of the lamina propria; and the 'body' which includes the stiffer vocal ligament and muscle layers. It has become evident that more than two mechanical layers may need to be accounted for to thoroughly explain vibratory phenomena. For example, the vocal ligament may serve as a biomechanical transition region, since its stiffness is intermediate between the cover and the muscle.

The degree to which the different vocal fold layers function separately during phonation depends on the action of intrinsic, and to some extent, extrinsic muscles of the larynx, as well as the health of vocal fold structures. In general terms, muscle groups that serve to lengthen and stiffen the mechanical layers make them function more as if they were one. This is the case during phonation at very high frequencies, as for example, in the loft or falsetto register. Disease processes affecting the cover may also serve to unify the function of the layers: edema in Reinke's space increases its viscosity, and results in less complex patterns of vibration; and surgical scarring may result in 'tethering' of the cover to the body. Muscles that tend to adduct the vocal folds without concurrent increases in muscular tone of the body may result in the two layers functioning more-or-less as if they were one, but in a very different manner than in the tense state. The acoustic result may include a degree of 'breathiness' (due to a lowered resistance to airflow, and subsequent longer open phase of the phonatory cycle). Denervation of the vocalis/thyro-arytenoid muscle, may result in reduced tone and viscosity of the body, and mechanical properties more similar to those of the cover. This is often noted in the case of vocal fold paralyses. Contraction of the vocalis/thyro-arytenoid muscle group, without a proportional increase in opposing lengthening forces (cricothyroid muscle), will make the body stiffer and the cover looser. This relatively looser cover is the situation in 'chest' or modal register, which is the usual speaking-voice register.

A frontal view of the vocal folds during one phonatory cycle in modal register is represented schematically in Figure 10.10. At least four distinct vocal fold shapes may be represented in the phonatory cycle in modal register: convergent; sulcus; rectangular; and divergent [12, 42, 55], with the definitions based largely on the nature of vertical phase differences between the upper and lower margins of the vocal folds. Scherer and Titze [42] have demonstrated how each of these shapes must be associated with a different set of aerodynamic and mechanical principles. Of particular importance during the vibratory cycle is the divergent shape associated with the onset of closing phase. In the past, the aerodynamic aspect of vocal fold self-oscillation focused exclusively on the **Bernoulli principle** thought to be the primary aerodynamic restoring force for the vocal fold closing phase [58]. The predominant closing influence of this principle depends on an assumption of laminar (smooth, non-turbulent) symmetrical airflow through a rectangular-shaped glottis. It is now clear that the divergent shape of vocal fold closing in modal register must result in other important non-symmetrical aerodynamic principles contributing to vocal fold closure, principally **flow separation**: separation of the airstream from its boundary at the glottic outlet, associated with turbulence [27]. Further, differential and interacting aerodynamic forces

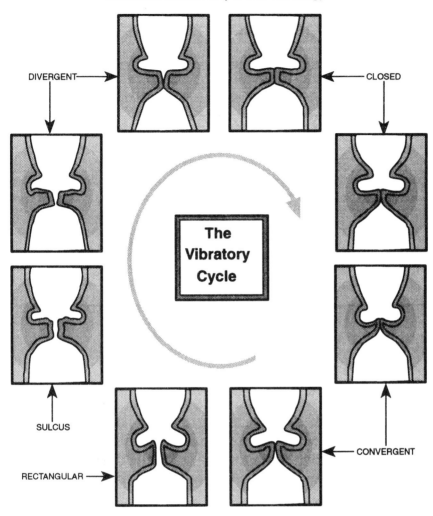

DIVERGENT

CLOSED

The
Vibratory
Cycle

SULCUS

RECTANGULAR

CONVERGENT

Figure 10.10 Frontal view of one phonatory cycle in modal register. Four different glottic shapes are represented, corresponding to at least four different aerodynamic principles that may be in effect during phonation in this register.

are present at different levels of the glottis throughout the phonatory cycle, and these depend on the shapes the vocal folds assume at any one time, as influenced by the amplitude, frequency and register of the vibration [26, 50–52].

Phonation in other registers: falsetto or glottal fry are associated with shapes and biomechanical principles that are quite different from those for modal register. For example, in falsetto singing register, the vocal fold cover is stiffened considerably by anteroposterior lengthening, so the layers function more like one. The vocal fold margins are much thinner in the superior–inferior dimension, which affects other aspects of vocal fold vibration to be discussed in the following paragraphs. Finally, reduced contraction of the thyro-arytenoid muscles may reduce myo-elastic vocal fold adduction properties, so the closed phase of phonation may be incomplete or of short duration. In glottal fry or pulse register, the cover may be loose and the body stiff as with modal register, but the closed phase of the vibratory cycle is proportionally longer, suggesting some other muscular forces are creating anterior–posterior constriction and medial compression.

An important consequence of the multiple-layer structure is the potential for a very complex vibratory pattern of the vocal folds. A number of dynamic phenomena may be partially explainable on the basis of the variable layer structure: **longitudinal phase difference**, **vertical phase difference**, and **mucosal wave**. These three effects are particularly noticeable in modal or chest register phonation, and together determine the potential for a complex sound wave with many harmonic components.

Longitudinal phase difference

Longitudinal phase difference refers to nonsimultaneous opening and closing of different portions of the vocal folds in the anterior to posterior direction, giving a zipper-type opening and closing effect. The longitudinal phase difference may be a consequence of: variable thicknesses of the different layers from anterior to posterior; variable muscular dynamics from anterior to posterior; different nature of structural attachments of the anterior and posterior portions of the vocal folds; and differential mechanical and aerodynamic consequences of all the above factors, from anterior to posterior.

Vertical phase difference

Vertical phase difference relates to temporal differences in the opening and closing of the bottom and top margins of the vocal folds. In modal register, the vocal folds open and close from the inferior to superior margins. Since the inferior margins are subjected to subglottic pressures first, the vertical phase difference is easily explainable on the basis of upward-flowing aerodynamic forces and a mechanical linkage dragging the superior edges in the direction of the inferior edges. The inertial elastic forces of the stretched vocal fold tissues, along with any relevant aerodynamic forces, effect the closing phases of the cycle beginning at the lower margins, and mechanically drag the upper margins with some phase lag.

Mucosal wave

Mucosal wave is the ripple effect seen along the surface of the vocal folds: a ripple that stretches more or less from the anterior to posterior ends, and travels from the margin to the peripheral area of each of the vocal folds. It is thought to be related to several factors including the vertical phase difference, and the natural tendency for the mechanical cover to move freely when the incompressible vocal folds are subjected to vertical deformation by subglottic pressures. Additional factors that may influence the mucosal wave include the impact between the vocal folds when they collide, and reflections from the lateral ventricle walls. It has been revealed that the velocity of the propagation of mucosal waves influences the phase lag between the upper and lower vocal fold margins.

It should be evident that vibration of the vocal folds during phonation is due to both aerodynamic and mechanical principles. The potential for maintaining vibration is dependent on a complex interaction between asymmetrical aerodynamic and mechanical forces. Broad [5] has described this relationship succinctly: 'Vibrations can be sustained only if the effective aerodynamic coupling between the glottic outlet and inlet is stronger than the mechanical coupling between the corresponding upper and lower parts of the vocal fold'. The relative influence of aerodynamic and mechanical forces may be determined by vocal production factors such as vocal effort or tension and pitch. Phonation at high pitches is associated with more symmetrical vocal fold margins, and smaller vertical phase differences.

Titze [53, 54] has studied phonation threshold pressures for different vocal production conditions. These studies suggest that phonation at lower fundamental frequencies is more responsive to aerodynamic forces than phonation at higher f_0 levels. That is, phonation can be initiated and sustained with lower subglottic pressures when the vocal folds are in their shorter, thicker state as in the modal speech register. The interactions and relative contributions of aerodynamic and mechanical forces in vocal fold vibration are also influenced by amplitude of the vibrations, and posturing factors such as degree of adduction of the arytenoid cartilages. The infinite possibilities for different vocal fold vibratory patterns and resultant acoustic products are far from understood at this time. Some recent studies using animal and computer models present the complexity of issues that must be addressed before we can understand vocal fold vibratory patterns [1, 16, 27, 39, 50, 55–57].

10.4.2 Dynamic Control of Pitch, Intensity and Quality

During speech, the intrinsic muscles of the larynx function in complex ways to continuously alter the frequency, amplitude, and pattern of vibration, therefore causing changes to acoustic and perceptual features of voice: pitch, loudness, and quality. The degree to which elastic tissue properties versus aerodynamic features contribute to changes in f_0 and intensity may depend on the phonatory register (mode of vibration), technique, articulatory resistance in the vocal tract, and even motivational and emotional factors.

Intrinsic muscles that are involved in various pitch and intensity-changing functions are represented in Figure 10.11.

Within modal register, changes in the fundamental frequency of vibration are due primarily to changes in the stiffness or tension of the vocal folds. The cricothyroid muscles contract to adjust the distance between the two cartilage structures, thus lengthening and stiffening the vocal folds. The effectiveness of cricothyroid contraction

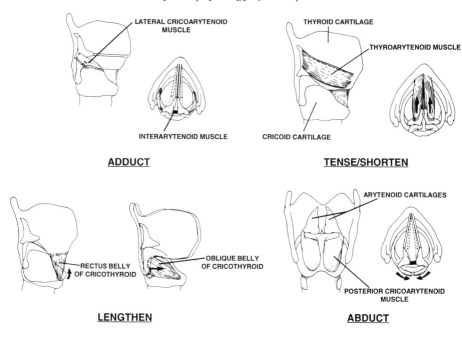

Figure 10.11 Intrinsic muscles in the larynx and their primary functions for phonation.

in achieving this task is dependent on opposing contraction of adducting (and sometimes abducting) muscles that anchor the arytenoid cartilages. Concurrent contraction of the vocalis/thyro-arytenoid complex helps to increase tension to contribute to pitch increases, particularly in the modal register. Mechanisms for pitch lowering seem to be primarily related to cessation of activity in the muscles that increase f_0. In studies of speech intonation, both aerodynamic forces and larynx lowering by action of extrinsic muscles have also been implicated in pitch lowering mechanisms [3, 6]. Differential intonation mechanisms may be used at low versus high pitch ranges for speech, and also mechanisms may differ based on syntactic characteristics of speech (sentence type) [3]. Clearly many questions need to be answered before we fully understand relationships between linguistic and physiological aspects of intonation control. Under certain conditions, such as phonation in falsetto register, aerodynamic forces may play a greater role in effecting f_0 variation because small amplitudes of vibration determine amplitude-dependent f_0 changes [52, 53, 55, 56]. These forces may be influenced by properties of the sub- and supraglottic cavities that influence aerodynamics during phonation.

Vocal intensity is primarily a function of subglottic pressure and amplitude of vocal fold vibrations, however the vocal tract filter function and radiation characteristic of speech also influence the intensity of the final speech product. Acoustic intensity is proportional to subglottic pressure, which you will remember, is determined by airflow and glottic resistance. Rapid changes in intensity are required to provide linguistic stress, and as we have discussed, the achievement of these linguistic markers involves complex interactions between laryngeal valving forces and aerodynamic driving forces.

Voice quality is related both to individual structural/mechanical features and to habitual laryngeal and supraglottic postures. Let us look at a graphic representation of the glottic pulse to explore some possible physiological correlates of voice quality. In Figure 10.12 one cycle of vocal fold oscillation in modal register is represented by a single glottic pulse, as seen in a flow glottogram. We see that normal phonation in modal register is associated with a skewed waveform. A more gradual slope in the opening phase suggests that the vocal folds open relatively slower, and a steeper slope in the closing phase suggests they close relatively faster. This skewed pulse is more noticeable in the average adult male voice than adult female voice, likely for structural and physiological reasons. The faster closing phase of phonation has been related to an acoustic signal that is relatively rich in harmonic components of the waveform and especially those that enhance the important speech and singing formants of the upper vocal tract as seen in Figure 10.13a [45]. If the length of the closing phase is increased

The Glottal Pulse

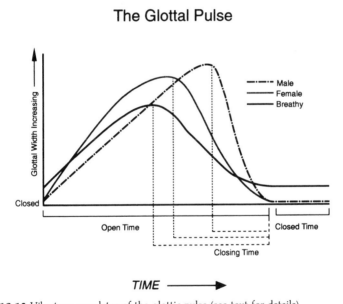

Figure 10.12 Vibratory correlates of the glottic pulse (see text for details).

(open phase increases) then the vocal 'sound' may not be so clear due to relatively lower amplitude of the upper harmonics and formants of the voice, as seen in Figure 10.13b [39]. The consensus that some North American women have 'breathier' voices than do men may be related to the slower closing phase in phonation. This voice quality and vibratory feature may also be related to presence of a posterior glottic chink, which has been identified as a frequent characteristic of phonatory posturing in women. Phonation

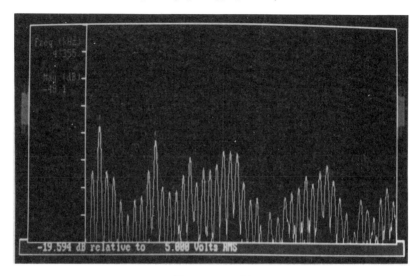

Figure 10.13 (a)

with a large posterior glottic chink may result in excessive noise in the vocal signal, where harmonics are replaced by air turbulence, and a noise peak may be seen in the upper vocal spectrum. [40, 43] As well, the relative intensity of f_0, the first harmonic partial of the glottic source acoustic waveform, may be greater than that of the other areas of the spectrum [31, 40]. These phenomena are demonstrated in Figure 10.13c. Such an acoustic profile generally results in perceptions of 'breathiness'. The schematic glottic pulse for a clinically breathy voice is seen in Figure 10.12 as the most symmetrical waveform.

'Harsh' or 'rough' qualities have been attributed to irregularities or perturbations in consecutive vibratory cycles, resulting in 'jitter' (irregular durations of cycles); and 'shimmer' (irregular amplitudes of cycles) in the acoustic waveform [7, 38, 49]. Figure 10.14 demonstrates these perturbations in the glottic source waveform schematically.

Extrinsic muscles also make many adjustments which may contribute to perceptual changes in the voice (Figure 10.15). For example, unopposed contraction of suprahyoid muscles will cause the larynx to rise in the neck, and may elevate pitch by increasing vocal fold tension, and secondarily by shortening the resonance tube, thus elevating vocal tract resonances or **formants** [8]. If extrinsic muscle activity has an influence on vocal fold tension and adduction, then voice quality may be affected further. Conversely, larynx lowering may result in reduced vocal fold tension to lower fundamental frequency, and a longer vocal tract to lower formants and pitch.

Any long-term postures in muscles of the pharynx, velopharynx or articulators, can influence speech or voice quality perceptions further. For example: the relative degree to which the tongue is held forward or back in the mouth during speech will influence resonance and articulatory qualities; the relative degree to which the jaw is held fixed, or is mobile during speech will influence oral/nasal resonance balance; and the degree to

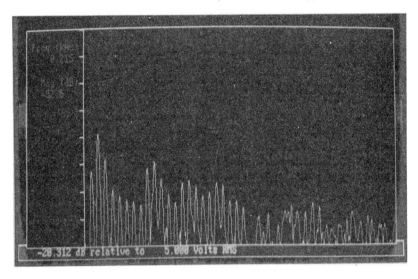

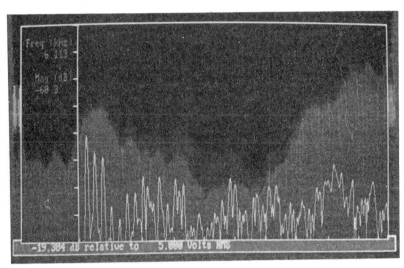

Figure 10.13 Characteristics of the vibratory pattern contribute to spectral features in the speech waveform pattern, or spectrum. In each spectrum, the abscissa represents frequency and the ordinate intensity. (a) Intensity-enhanced, high-frequency harmonics (vertical lines) and speech formants (envelop) are represented by relative height. Rapid vocal fold closure contributes to greater intensities in the high-frequency portion of the speech waveform; (b) longer duration of the vocal fold closing phase contributes to lower intensity in the high frequency portion of the speech waveform; (c) phonation with large glottic chinks is associated with a relatively high intensity in the fundamental (first harmonic partial is the first vertical line on the left) and noise in the spectrum. The noise may be particularly intense in the region above 5 kHz. These acoustic characteristics may contribute to perceptions of 'breathiness' or 'whisperiness'.

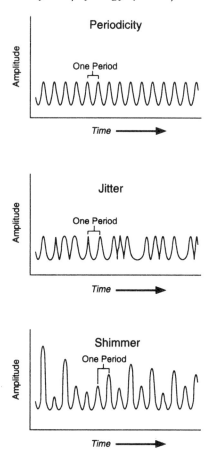

Figure 10.14 Variations or perturbations in the glottic source waveform may contribute to acoustic characteristics such as jitter and shimmer. In reality, absolute periodicity is not a common feature of phonatory activity for speech.

which the velopharyngeal port is closed or open will determine the perceived 'nasality' [32, 33].

10.5 ACOUSTIC RESONATORS OF SPEECH

Figure 10.16 shows the structures involved in vocal tract resonance. Figure 10.17 demonstrates the fundamental principles of acoustic waveform transformations during speech. As the glottic pulse propagates along the vocal tract it is subjected to a variety of resonance effects that are determined by the shape and viscosity of the cavity walls. The principles are based on the *Acoustic Theory of Speech Production* proposed by Fant [8].

The original acoustic theory describes relationships between the glottic source features, vocal tract filter function and radiation characteristics.

The **glottic source** contributes a fairly regular pulse-like multi-frequency input signal to the vocal tract. In the case of an ideal periodic voice source input signal, the frequencies represented in the glottic pulse are mathematically predictable: the strongest component will correspond to the fundamental frequency and progressively weaker components or harmonic partials fall at frequencies corresponding to $f_0 \times 2$; $f_0 \times 3$; $f_0 \times 4$ .... An amplitude density spectrum demonstrates that the intensity of progressively higher harmonic partials is reduced by about 12 dB per octave, when source characteristics are considered independent of the vocal tract filter function. In reality, vocal sounds are not perfectly harmonic, and even in normal speech the vocal source waveform may be characterized by minor perturbations (irregularities) and areas of noise energy. These normal variations from idealized glottic pulses, in addition to the vocal tract filter functions, influence the harmonic energy patterns in speech spectra.

The vocal tract characteristics serve to enhance or dampen various frequency components, or groups of adjacent partials of the glottic pulse waveform. Positioning of the articulators, including the larynx and cavity walls, result in distinct shapes of the vocal tract corresponding to specific natural resonance characteristics, called formants. The first two or three formants (and antiformants) can be used to predict and describe articulatory features for continuous sounds of a language, for example the vowel

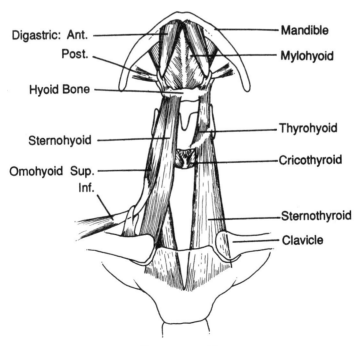

Figure 10.15 (a)

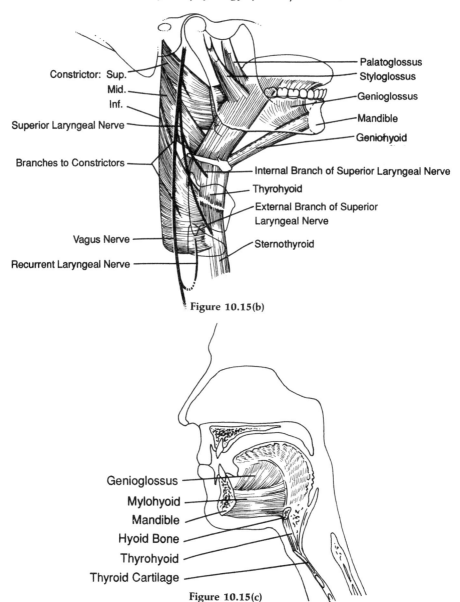

Figure 10.15(b)

Figure 10.15(c)

Figure 10.15 Structure and muscles of the larynx. The supralaryngeal and infralaryngeal muscles suspend the larynx in the neck and may be active during changes in vocal intensity, frequency or resonance characteristics. When hypertonic, these muscles in various combinations may contribute to limitations in phonatory function, and dysphonia. (a) Frontal view demonstrating extrinsic muscle larynx suspension system; (b) lateral view demonstrating relationships of pharyngeal muscles with the larynx, and nerve supply; (c) lateral view demonstrating relationships of tongue and mandible muscles with the larynx.

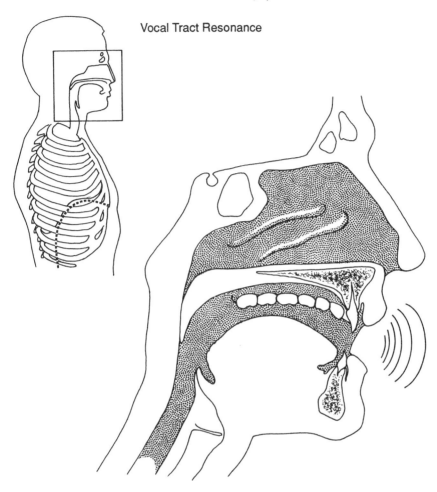

Vocal Tract Resonance

Figure 10.16 Vocal tract resonators for speech are primarily the upper larynx, pharynx and oral cavities. The nasal cavities contribute resonance characteristics when the velopharyngeal port is open, most obviously for nasal phonemes /m/; /n/; /ŋ/.

phonemes. The frequencies of formants can be predicted within a certain range for particular vocal tract lengths: for example the average formants for North American English /i/ are F_1: 270 Hz; F_2: 2300 Hz; F_3: 3000 Hz for an adult male, and F_1: 370 Hz; F_2: 3200 Hz and F_3: 3700 Hz for a preschool child [29]. During speech the formants are in almost constant transition, and often do not reach the precise values that predict sound discriminations, owing to continual movement of the articulators and co-articulatory effects. Even in the brief time that is allotted to a series of speech targets, acoustic filter functions provide the listener with sufficient formant information and other important

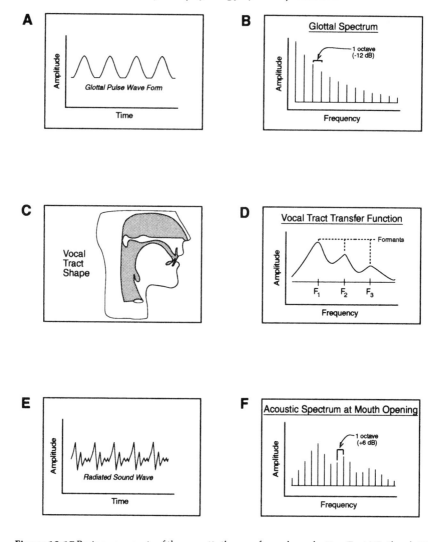

Figure 10.17 Basic components of the acoustic theory of speech production (Fant [8]): the glottic pulse (A and B); vocal tract transfer function (C and D); and radiation characteristics (E and F) (see text for details).

acoustic cues to recognize speech. Figure 10.18 demonstrates schematically a lateral view of the vocal tract during production of three North American English vowels, and their corresponding vocal tract filter spectra.

A final important acoustic characteristic encompassed in Fant's theory is that of the **radiation characteristic** of speech. This function describes the nature of propagation of the speech sounds through the air from the end of the vocal tract, and further defines the nature of sound that reaches the listener's ear. The radiation characteristic can be

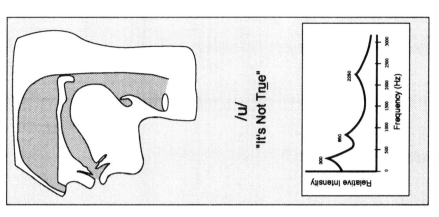

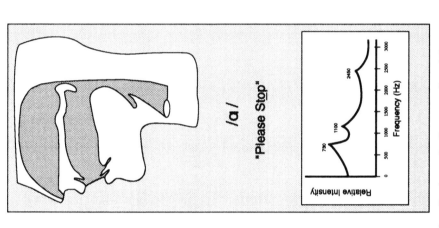

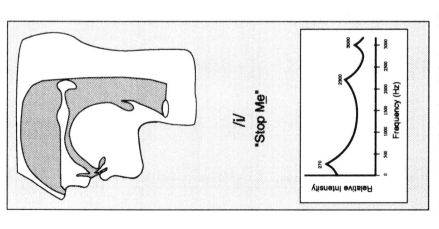

Figure 10.18 Idealized sagittal views of the oral cavity shapes for three vowels and their corresponding speech formants.

predicted to increase the speech signal by 6 dB per octave. This feature seems to coincide with the sensitivity of the human acoustic system.

Although the original acoustic theory of speech has provided a valuable reference for descriptions of speech function in an idealized fashion, its simplicity limits description of certain aspects of normal and disordered speech function. For example, interactions between the glottic source function and vocal tract adjustments may influence the nature of the final radiated acoustic signal, due to mechanical aerodynamic loading forces, and acoustic interactions. Further, the supraglottic and subglottic spaces may be coupled to varying degrees during speech and phonation, depending on the length of open phases in the phonatory cycle, and the degree of approximation of the vocal folds [9–11, 41, 46].

10.6 NORMAL VARIABILITY IN STRUCTURE AND FUNCTION

A wide range of anatomical and functional variability of the human voice has been documented. Even within sexes, age groups and body types, one must consider the norm to be a continuum with fuzzy boundaries. This includes, size, shape, and vibratory characteristics of the larynx; psycho-acoustic and acoustic parameters such as pitch range, loudness range, and quality; sound-wave perturbations; and other relevant dynamics such as phonatory airflow rate and subglottic pressure. Normative data is constantly being collected and analysed in clinics across the globe, but for many parameters no consensus has been reached as to where normal ends and abnormal begins.

10.6.1 Normal Development and Aging

In the infant, the larynx is positioned differently than in the adult, and structural development is incomplete. The larynx is high in the neck at birth (the cricoid cartilage rests between C2 and C3 of the cervical vertebrae) and positioned thus, tucked under the tongue, the infant is able to alternate rapidly between suckling and breathing without aspirating. The opening to the larynx is narrow, due to the shape of cartilages in infancy. The hyoid bone and thyroid cartilage function as one, and the cartilage structure in general is much more flexible. The vocal fold layer structure is much simpler than in the adult: newborns have very thick mucosal layers, and there is no vocal ligament apparent, rather a uniform lamina propria structure more like that of the superficial layer (Reinke's space) in adults. [15]. Histological studies have suggested that in the infant, laryngeal muscles have fewer type 1 muscles: those known to have slow and prolonged contraction, than do adults. One possible function served by a large proportion of type 2 muscles in infants is effective and rapid opening and closing of the glottis to allow for rapid inspiration without aspiration during feeding [30].

In older children and adults, a larger proportion of type 1 muscle fibers in laryngeal muscles may assist in more refined laryngeal gestures, and prolonged vocal fold adduction for the purposes of verbal communication. The formation of a poorly differentiated vocal ligament begins in the preschool years, and two layers become apparent before puberty. Articulatory structures as well, are not fully developed at birth. In particular, muscle coordination and strength of the tongue is inferior to that of adults. Nevertheless, the infant is capable of producing a wide-enough repertoire of vocal sounds for selective communication to occur: mothers quickly learn to distinguish among the various cries, to oblige the appropriate requests.

At puberty, a sex differentiation is realized in the nature and degree of many aspects of vocal development. By the end of puberty, the larynx has assumed a lower position in the neck, where it rests between C6 and C7 of the cervical vertebrae. In concert with other growth spurts, the larynx of males virtually doubles in size, usually in a short period of a few months, with increases in neck and vocal tract sizes usually preceding or concurrent. The overall effect is a dramatic drop in the natural fundamental frequency range of vibration: usually at least a one octave change. In addition, because the resonance chamber increases in length and width, the formant frequencies drop, to contribute further to a 'deep', masculine voice. The angle of the thyroid cartilage has decreased from 120° to about 90° in the mature male larynx. The epiglottis may change shape, becoming less omega-shaped. Hirano has suggested that male and female adolescents have developed full vocal ligaments by age 15 [15]. The growth of the female larynx during puberty is much slower and less dramatic, and may continue into the early 20s. The angle of the thyroid cartilage does not change significantly, and although both the larynx and vocal tract increase in size, the overall pitch and resonance changes are less than in the male. In addition to differences in overall size differences, gender-based differences in the shape of the vocal tract have been reported in the adolescent larynx. In men, the pharynx grows proportionally larger than the oral cavity, compared with vocal tract maturation processes in women [28, 29].

Some developmental differences, as identified during laryngoscopy and histology, are represented in Figure 10.19.

Several changes in laryngeal and vocal tract structure and histology may contribute to the sound of the 'aged voice'. Again, some of the changes and schedules tend to be different for men and women. In the male larynx, histological changes may be noted in the fourth decade, whereas female aging signs do not generally appear until the fifth decade of life. Changes in the male larynx include muscle atrophy, reduced elasticity, and fibrotic changes in the elastic and collagen layers of the lamina propria. Reductions in bulk, muscle tone, and elasticity may explain a tendency for the natural fundamental frequency of the male to rise in later years. (Some may resist the change by pushing the larynx lower, speaking in glottic fry register, or otherwise compensating muscularly). In the female, atrophic changes may be less significant, but greater bulk of the vocal folds often results from increased edema in the superficial layer of the lamina propria. The overall effect on phonation is to produce a potentially lower fundamental frequency of vibration. Females may resist the change to a more 'masculine' tone, by tensing muscles, raising the larynx, etc. In addition to these sex-specific changes, characteristics of the aging voice can be influenced by systemic diseases, such as arthritis, respiratory ailments, and neuromuscular diseases, such as dysarthria, parkinsonism and tremors. Voice changes related to aging and disease processes in the elderly are discussed in

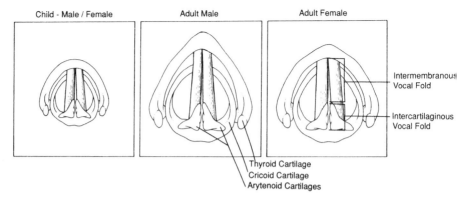

Figure 10.19 Structural differences for adults and children. (a) The proportion of cartilaginous glottis decreases after puberty, particularly evident in the male adult. The angle of the thyroid cartilage decreases in the male adult at puberty; (b) Histological development in the vocal fold. The newborn has a poorly differentiated layer structure, with no obvious vocal ligament. The origins of the anterior and posterior macula flava may represent the developing ligament. The full layer structure is not evident until age 12 or later. (After Hirano and Kurita [15], with permission.)

more detail in Chapter 8. The reader is also referred to additional reading on these topics [2, 14–16, 28, 30].

In summary, voice production plays an important role in verbal discourse, by providing an acoustic signal that makes speech audible. This signal is characterized by rapid or longer-term alterations in pitch, intensity, quality and duration that convey changes in emotion, meaning, and grammar.

The production of voice for speech requires complex and dynamic interactions among several anatomic and physiological systems. Members of the professional voice care team must be knowledgeable about structural and functional aspects of the complex voice production systems in order to formulate accurate diagnoses and develop appropriate treatment plans.

References

1. Alipour-Haghighi F. and Titze I.R. (1991) Elastic models of vocal fold tissues. *NCVS Status and Progress Report-1*, 39–48.
2. Aronson, A.E. (1985) *Clinical Voice Disorders*. Thieme, New York, NY.
3. Atkinson J.E. (1978) Correlation analysis of the physiological factors controlling fundamental voice frequency. *Journal of the Acoustic Society of America*, **63**, 211–22.
4. Baken R.J. (1987) *Clinical Measurement of Speech and Voice*. College-Hill, Boston, MA.
5. Broad D.J. (1979) The new theories of vocal fold vibration, in *Speech and Language: Advances in Basic Research and Practice*, Vol. 2 (ed. N.J. Lass), Academic, New York, pp. 203–55.
6. Collier R. (1975) Physiological correlates of intonation patterns. *Journal of the Acoustic Society of America*, **58**, 249–55.

Adult

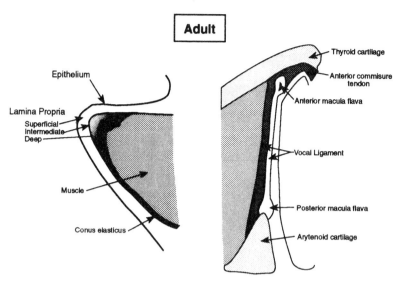

Infant

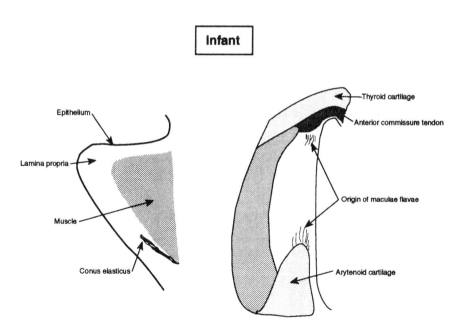

Figure 10.19 (b)

7. Davis S.B. (1979) Acoustic characteristics of normal and pathological voices, in *Speech and Language: Advances in Basic Research and Practice*, Vol 1. Academic, New York.

8. Fant G. (1960) *Acoustic Theory of Speech Production*, Mouton, The Hague.

9. Fant G. (1983) The voice source-theory and acoustic modelling, in *Vocal Fold Physiology: Biomechanics, Acoustics and Phonatory Control* (eds I.R. Titze and R.C. Scherer), Denver Center for the Performing Arts, Denver, CO.

10. Fant G. (1986) Glottal flow: models and interaction. *Journal of Phonetics*, **14**, 393–9.

11. Fant G. and Lin Q. (1991) Comments on glottal flow modelling and analysis, in *Vocal Fold Physiology: Acoustic, Perceptual and Physiological Aspects of Voice Mechanisms* (eds J. Gauffin and B. Hammarberg), Singular, San Diego, CA.

12. Hirano M. (1977) Structure and vibratory behavior of the vocal folds, in *Dynamic Aspects of Speech Production* (eds M. Sawashima and F.S. Cooper), University of Tokyo Press, Tokyo, pp. 13–27.

13. Hirano M. (1981) *Clinical Examination of Voice*. Springer-Verlag, New York.

14. Hirano M. (1983) Structure of the vocal fold in normal and disease states Anatomical and physical studies, in *Proceedings of the Conference on the Assessment of Vocal Pathology, ASHA Reports 11*, American Speech–Language–Hearing Association, Rockville, MD.

15. Hirano M. and Kurita S. (1986) Histological structure of the vocal fold and its normal and pathological variations, in *Vocal Fold Histopathology* (ed. J.A. Kirschner) College-Hill, Boston MA, pp. 17–24.

16. Hirano M., Kakita Y., Ohmaru K. and Kurita S. (1982) Structure and mechanical properties of the vocal fold, in *Speech and Language: Advances in Basic Research and Practice*, Vol. 7 (ed N.J. Lass), Academic, New York, pp. 271–97.

17. Hixon T.J. et al (1987) *Respiratory Function in Speech and Song*. Williams & Wilkins, Baltimore, MD.

18. Hixon T.J., Goldman M.D. and Mead J. (1973) Kinematics of the chest wall during speech production: volume displacements of the rib cage, abdomen, and lung. *Journal of Speech and Hearing Research* **16**(1) 78–115.

19. Hixon T.J., Mead J. and Goldman M.D. (1976) Dynamics of the chest wall during speech production: function of the thorax, rib cage, diaphragm, and abdomen. *Journal of Speech and Hearing Research*, **19**(2) 297–356.

20. Hixon T.J., Watson P.J. and Maher M.Z. (1987) Respiratory kinematics in classical (Shakespearean) actors, in *Respiratory Function in Speech and Song* (eds T.J. Hixon *et al.*) College-Hill, Boston, MA.

21. Hixon T.J., Watson P.J., Harris F.P. and Perlman N.B. (1988) Relative volume changes of the rib cage and abdomen during prephonatory chest wall posturing. *Journal of Voice*, **2**(1) 13–19.

22. Hodge M.M. and Putnam Rochet A. (1989) Characteristics of speech-breathing in young women. *Journal of Speech and Hearing Research*, **32**(3) 466–80.

23. Hoit J.D. and Hixon T.J. (1986) Body type and speech-breathing. *Journal of Speech and Hearing Research*, **29**(3) 313–24.

24. Hoit J.D. and Hixon T.J. (1987) Age and speech-breathing. *Journal of Speech and Hearing Research*, **30**(3) 351–66.

25. Hoit J.D., Hixon T.J., Altman M.E. and Morgan W.J. (1989) Speech-breathing in women. *Journal of Speech and Hearing Research*, **32**(2) 353–65.

26. Ishizaka K. and Flanagan J.L. (1977) Acoustic properties of longitudinal displacement in vocal fold vibration. *Bell System Technical Journal*, **56**, 889–918.

27. Ishizaka K. and Matsudaira M. (1972) Fluid mechanical considerations of vocal fold vibration. *SCRL Monograph No. 8*.

28. Kahane J.C. (1983) Postnatal development and aging of the human larynx. *Seminars in Speech and Language* **4**(3) 189–203.

29. Kent R.D. and Read C. (1992) *The Acoustic Analysis of Speech*. Singular, San Diego, CA.

30. Kersing W. (1986) Vocal musculature, aging and developmental aspects, in *Vocal Fold Histopathology* (ed. J.A. Kirchner), College-Hill, Boston MA, pp. 11–16.
31. Klatt D.H. and Klatt L.C. (1990) Analysis, synthesis, and perception of voice quality variations among female and male talkers. *Journal of the Acoustic Society of America*, **87**(2) 820–57.
32. Laver J. (1980) *The Phonetic Description of Voice Quality*, Cambridge University Press, Cambridge.
33. Laver J. (1991) *Vocal Profile Analysis*, University of Edinburgh, Edinburgh.
34. Leanderson R., Sundberg J. and von Euler C. (1984) Effects of diaphragm activity on phonation during singing. *Transcripts of the Thirteenth Symposium on Care of the Professional Voice*, Voice Foundation, New York, NY.
35. Leanderson R., Sundberg J., von Euler C. and Lagercrantz (1983) Diaphragmatic control of the subglottic pressure during singing. *Transcripts of the Twelfth Symposium on Care of the Professional Voice*, Voice Foundation, New York, NY.
36. Leinonen L. and Laakso M-L. (1990) Control of static pressure by expiratory muscles during expiratory effort and phonation. *Journal of Voice*, **4**(3) 256–63.
37. McFarland D.H. and Smith A. (1989) Surface recordings of respiratory muscle activity during speech: some preliminary findings. *Journal of Speech and Hearing Research*, **32**(3) 657–67.
38. Moore G.P. (1971) *Organic Voice Disorders*. Prentice-Hall, Englewood Cliffs, NJ.
39. Perlman A.L. and Durham P.L. (1987) In vitro studies of vocal fold mucosa during isometric conditions, in *Laryngeal Function in Phonation and Respiration (eds T. Baer, C. Sasaki and K. Hernis)*, College-Hill, Boston MA, pp. 291–303.
40. Rammage L.A. (1992) Acoustic, aerodynamic and stroboscopic characteristics of phonation with variable posterior glottis postures. Doctoral dissertation, University of Wisconsin-Madison.
41. Rothenberg M. (1983) Source-tract interaction in breathy voice, in *Vocal Fold Physiology: Biomechanics, Acoustics and Phonatory Control* (eds I.R. Titze and R.C. Scherer), Denver Center for the Performing Arts, Denver, CO.
42. Scherer R.C. and Titze I.R. (1981) A new look at van den Berg's glottal aerodynamics. *Transcripts of the Tenth Symposium on Care of the Professional Voice*, Voice Foundation, New York, NY.
43. Shoji K., Regenbogen E., Yu J.D. and Blaugrund S.M. (1992) High-frequency power ratio of breathy voice. *Laryngoscope*, **102**, 267–71.
44. Sundberg J. (1990) What's so special about singers? *Journal of Voice*, **4**(2) 107–19.
45. Sundberg J. (1987) *The Science of the Singing Voice*, Northern Illinois University, Dekalb, IL.
46. Sundberg J. and Askenfelt (1983) Larynx height and voice source: A relationship?, in *Vocal Fold Physiology: Contemporary Research and Clinical Issues* (eds D.M. Bless and J.H. Abbs), College-Hill, San Diego, CA.
47. Sundberg J., Leanderson R. and von Euler C. (1984) Effects of diaphragm activity on phonation during singing. *Transcripts of the Thirteenth Sypmposium on Care of the Professional Voice*, Voice Foundation, New York, NY.
48. Sundberg J., Leanderson R., von Euler C. and Knutsson E. (1991) Influence of body posture and lung volume on subglottal pressure control during singing. *Journal of Voice*, **5**(4) 283–91.
49. Takahashi H. and Koike Y. (1975) Some perceptual dimensions and acoustic correlates of pathologic voices. *Acta Otolaryngological*, **338** (Suppl.), 1–24.
50. Titze I.R. (1973) The human vocal cords: A mathematical model. Part I, *Phonetica*, **28**, 129–70
51. Titze I.R. (1974) The human vocal cords: A mathematical model. Part II, *Phonetica*, **29**, 1–21.
52. Titze I.R. (1980) Comments on the myoelastic-aerodynamic theory of phonation. *Journal of Speeched Hearing Researched*, **23**, 495–510.
53. Titze I.R. (1988) The physics of small-amplitude oscillation of the vocal folds. *Journal of the Acoustic Society of America*, **83**(4), 1536–52.
54. Titze I.R. Phonation threshold pressure. *Journal of the Acoustic Society of America* (in press).

55. Titze I.R. and Strong WJ (1975) Normal modes in vocal cord tissues. *Journal of the Acoustic Society of America*, **57**, 736–44.
56. Titze I.R. and Talkin D.T. (1979) A theoretical study of the effects of various laryngeal configurations on the acoustics of phonation. *Journal of the Acoustic Society of America*, **66**(1) 60–74.
57. Titze I.R., Jiang J. and Druker D.G. (1987) Preliminaries to the body-cover theory of pitch control. *Journal of Voice*, **1**(4), 314–19.
58. van den Berg J.W., Zantema J.T. and Doorenball P. Jr (1957) On the air resistance and the Bernoulli effect of the human larynx. *Journal of the Acoustic Society of America*, **29**, 626–31.
59. Watson P.J. and Hixon T.J. (1985) Respiratory kinematics in classical (opera) singers. *Journal of Speeched Hearing Research*, **28**(1) 104–22.
60. Watson P.J., Hixon T.J., Stathopoulos E.T. and Sullivan D.R. (1990) Respiratory kinematics in female classical singers. *Journal of Voice*, **4**(2) 120–8.
61. Watson P.J., Hoit J.D., Lansing R.W. and Hixon T.J. (1989) Abdominal muscle activity during classical singing. *Journal of Voice*, **3**(1) 24–31.
62. Weismer G. (1988) Speech production, in *Handbook of Speech, Language and Hearing Pathology* (eds N. Lass, L. McReynolds, J. Northern and D. Yoder), Mosby Year Book, St Louis, MO.
63. Wilder C.N. (1983) Chest wall preparation for phonation in female speakers, in *Vocal Fold Physiology*, (eds D.M. Bless and J.H. Abbs) College-Hill, San Diego, CA.

Further reading

Aronson, A.E. (1985) *Clinical Voice Disorders*, Thieme, New York, NY.
Baer H., Sasaki C. ed Harris K.S. (1985) *Laryngeal Function in Phonation and Respiration*, College-Hill, Baston, MA.
Baken R.J. (1987) *Clinical Measurement of Speech and Voice*, College-Hill, Boston, MA.
Bless D.M. ed Abbs J.H. (1983) *Vocal Fold Physiology: Contemporary and Research Issues.* College-Hill, San Diego, CA.
Folkins J. ed Kahane J. (1984) *Atlas of Speech and Hearing Anatomy*. Charles E. Merrill, Columbus, OH.
Fujimura O. (1988) *Vocal Physiology: Voice Production, Mechanisms and Functions*, Raven Press, New York, NY.
Gauffin J. ed Hammarberg B. (1991) *Vocal Fold Physiology: Acoustic, Perceptual, and Physiological Aspects of Voice Mechanisms*, Singular, San Diego, CA.
Hirano M, Kirchner J.A. ed Bless D.M. (1987) *Neurolaryngology: Recent Advances*, College-Hill, Boston, MA.
Hixon T. *et al.* (1987) *Respiratory Function in Speech and Song*. College-Hill, Boston, MA.
Kahane J.C. ed Folkins J.W. (1984) *Atlas of Speech and Hearing Anatomy* Charles E. Merrill, Columbus, OH.
Kirchner, J.A. (1986) *Vocal Fold Histopathology*, College Hill, Boston, MA.
Stevens K.N. ed Hirano M. (1981) *Vocal Fold Physiology*, University of Tokyo, Tokyo.
Sundberg J. (1987) *The Science of the Singing Voice*, Northern Illinois University, Dekalb, IL.
Titze I.R. (1993) *Vocal Fold Physiology: Frontiers in Basic Science*. Singular, San Diego, CA.
Titze I.R. ed Scherer R.C. (1983) *Vocal Fold Physiology: Biomechanics, Acoustics and Phonatory Control*, Denver Center for the Performing Arts, Deaver, CO.
Tucker H. (1987) *The Larynx*. Thieme Medical, New York, NY.
van den Berg, W. (1960) *The Vibrating Larynx* (videotape).
Warren D. (1988) Aerodynamics of speech, in *Handbook of Speech-Language Pathology and Audiology*, N.J. Lass, L.V. McReynolds, J.L. Northern, D.E. Yoder, B.C. Decker, ⊃???⊂
Weismer G. (1988) Speech production, in *Handbook of Speech, Language and Hearing Pathology*, N. Lass, L. McReynolds, J. Northern and D. Yoder, B.C. Decker, ???
Zemlin, Willard (1988) *Speech and Hearing Science*, 3rd edn, Prentice-Hall, Englewood Cliffs, NJ.

11

Basics of singing pedagogy

Every culture uses the singing voice and, although the mechanism is the same, the cultural traditions of voice production are as different as the faces, languages, and ceremonies of the peoples of the world. In the Western tradition of classical music, there are some broadly accepted norms of what makes good and bad singing, and what is 'healthy' and 'unhealthy' vocal behavior. Even within this tiny part of Western culture there is enormous disagreement about the details of vocal production, and singing teachers have the reputation of being unable to agree with each other unless they belong to the same 'school' of pedagogy. Before stating what is unequivocally 'right' in singing technique and how a voice teacher should go about achieving it, it is important to establish clear terms of reference. The 'correct' method about which singing teachers strive to find agreement is not that used for Chinese classical opera, native Indian traditional music, Tibetan monks chanting, and, above all, it is not right for the huge majority of music in Western (and increasingly Eastern) society, i.e., 'pop' music (rock and roll in its many manifestations).

It is important for any voice teacher to decide whether the primary objective of voice training is to produce a singer who is maximizing the potential of the voice, while gaining understanding of the process, or producing a series of slightly imperfect clones of the teacher's own voice. The teacher's aim should be to become redundant. The voice teacher is not dealing with a verifiable scientific experiment; there is no 'control,' because voices will develop in size and quality with increasing age and experience, even if nothing happens to interfere with the natural process. Most important, the teacher is rarely in the position to deal with what one might delicately call a 'vocal virgin'. Singers will always have sung before having lessons, and will have picked up along the way a complex amalgam of influences – from parental singing to the baby, to radio, TV – through a series of role models (often very diverse) – through choirs and other ensembles, all gradually establishing a vocal personality and technique of singing. Genetic, linguistic, and cultural factors also play an important part in establishing a pattern of vocal behavior.

In training the singing voice, some general rules can be applied:

- Singing should be perceived by the audience as a free and natural activity. Despite its mechanical and energy requirements singers must never display to their audience overt signs of the effort involved in the production and the sustaining of vocal tone.

- Singing must be practiced in the same way as other instruments, and singers must know what and why they are practising. Skills need time and perseverance for them to develop fully. From this investment of time and energy, singers should emerge with a solid vocal technique that will give them knowledgeable control over the mechanics and expressiveness of their voices.
- Vocal technique must never be an end in itself, however fascinating and engrossing the subject becomes. Singers are athletes, not body-builders. Music is, after all, what this is all about and most of us have had the experience of sitting through hours of technically well-schooled vocal production from a singer with no glimmer of musical intelligence or understanding. We have also been bowled over by a singer with some vocal problems, but great intensity and deep musical understanding.
- Singing teachers should never try to make silk purses out of sows' ears. Natural talent is the most important factor in determining the ultimate potential of a voice. All voices have their individual natural limitations and a teacher's primary goal should be to help singers to reach their own potential.

In the context of this book it is not possible nor appropriate to attempt to lay out a complete method of voice production. The world of voice pedagogy contains numerous conflicting ideas of how the singing voice works and how it should be trained. These views divide along both historic and nationalistic lines and a study of the existing literature reveals some weird and wonderful interpretations of the aforementioned physical and acoustical laws alongside some intelligent and insightful understanding. Despite the diversity of opinion, we believe that it is possible to set down some basic principles with which most teachers would probably agree and which form the basis of good, healthy voice production.

11.1 OVERVIEW OF THE VOCAL INSTRUMENT

It is generally acknowledged that, functioning under the direction of physiological and acoustical laws, the vocal instrument has respiratory, phonatory, resonance, and articulatory components, and that these specific functions can be assigned to certain anatomical parts of the instrument. The respiratory function is the power plant, consisting of the inhalatory–exhalatory system which is housed principally in the torso but also includes the airways of the mouth, nose, and throat. The vibrating system is housed in the larynx. The resonance system is made up of a series of adjustable cavities in the neck and the head that modify the laryngeal tone. The articulatory function takes place within the resonance system and involves the tongue, lips, teeth, and the cheeks, which modify the product into spoken language. The brain, of course, is the master of all these parts, and initiates and coordinates, or alternatively inhibits and disrupts, the functions that result in an acoustic signal we call the voice (Figure 11.1).

In order to produce the singing voice these systems must work interdependently, but it is sometimes necessary to be able to consider them separately. Before taking that particular step, however, it is important to understand clearly the manner in which the gross framework of the body is organized in space and how it deals with the stresses of

An Overview of the Vocal Instrument

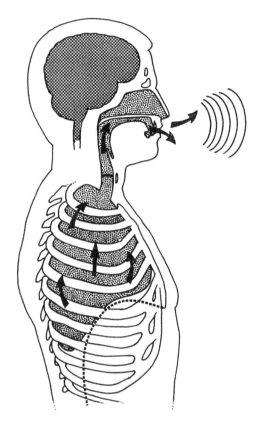

Figure 11.1 An overview of the vocal instrument.

gravity and everyday usage. In other words we are talking about matters that we usually think of as being related to posture.

11.2 POSTURE

It should be obvious that good posture is of central importance to good singing, yet it is often either neglected or curiously distorted. How we organize our bodies in space and how we habitually use them in daily life is in accordance with usage patterns that have evolved over the course of our lives. These patterns that we have developed since early childhood have usually grown, not from a careful consideration of the most efficient and effective way to carry out a specific physical task, but from a process that evolves as each task is accomplished. The goal of a child learning to walk is primarily one of establishing balance and then getting from A to B without falling over. Each task is pursued in a goal-orientated manner with no consideration of the quality of the action or the nature of the habit pattern that is being established. This process enables most people to sustain normal, active lives. It is only when we decide to pursue athletic or artistic activities that require high levels of skill, dexterity, and stamina, that a qualitative evaluation of the physical organization and usage patterns becomes necessary. Posture must provide, for the singer, the flexibility and freedom of movement that is essential to the singing instrument.

11.2.1 Predictable Faults in Postural Organization

There are many ways that the body can be arranged in the gravitational field, but for the singer, as with the athlete, it is convenient for us to think of the body in a standing, upright position. In this position there are predictable, organizational faults that can frequently be observed centered around the spine, its curvatures, and balance of the head.

It is not uncommon to observe the following postural faults:

* a forward collapse of the cervical vertebrae;
* a strong down-pull of the muscles of the back of the neck;
* the jaw jutted forward;
* an increase in the curvature of the dorsal spine;
* shoulders slumped forward and raised up towards the ears;
* a general narrowing of the back;
* a locking of the knees and a fixing of the pelvis in a forward and downward tilted position;
* a side-to-side pelvic displacement;
* an uneven distribution of weight over the feet.

Figures 11.2 and 11.3 show good and poor postural alignments and head and neck displacements.

The effect of this is to cause an increase in the natural curvature of the lumbar spine and a forward thrust of the abdominal contents against a distended abdominal wall. The postural organization of most human beings contains some of the above mentioned faults, and these can become exaggerated by stress, fatigue, and cultural conditioning.

11.2.2 Posture and Singing Performance

Public performance is filled with stress and physical fatigue, further complicated by the need to create credible characterizations and emotional body language that is quite different from the performer's own nature. The singer who exhibits any of the above listed postural faults would find, when confronted by performance demands, that neck and jaw tension interferes with laryngeal and articulatory activity, and that the collapsing thoracic framework and lumbar spine severely restricts breathing activities. It is clear that in order to comply with the physical needs of transforming the body into a sophisticated musical instrument and of being able to maintain that instrument through

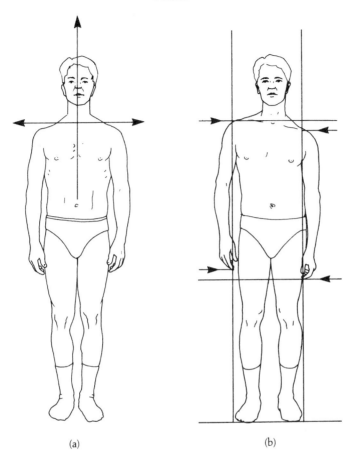

(a) (b)

Figure 11.2 Postural alignments and head and neck displacements in singing. (a) good posture, frontal view; (b) poor posture, frontal view.

the rigorous demands of a performing life, postural organization must not be left to the devices of habitual patterns that could lead to misuse.

One's posture is something that can be consciously organized and controlled, and any would-be singers must assume that responsibility if they hope to be successful. A thorough understanding of existing habit patterns and a knowledge of what must be readjusted in the best interests of singing is required. There is in singing, as in dance, and in most athletic activities a position of 'at the ready', of preparedness, the 'place' from which something muscular and coordinated can happen. This is not a fixed position but one of poise and balance from which easy movement can take place. The question is: 'How do we get there?'.

We learn from the work of F.M. Alexander that the key to all postural organization is the relationship that exists between the upper back, cervical vertebrae, shoulders, and balance of the head [1, 4]. The cruciform arrangement that exists at the top of the torso can, under pressure or misuse, collapse in on itself with contraction of the neck, slumping of the upper spine, narrowing of the back, and raising of the shoulders. Any realignment of posture must begin therefore with a series of mental directives that will lengthen the neck, widen the back, and release and widen the shoulders. This opening out allows the head to release, with a small nodding action, from its poked-forward attitude to a poised and balanced position on the top of the spine. From that position it is free to pivot easily as required. The sternum, as a result of the neck lengthening and shoulder widening, moves to a slightly raised position that gives the body a noble, elegant, ready look (Figure 11.3). The feeling is of a lengthened spine from which the ribs and thoracic musculature are free to respond to the demands of the respiratory system. The body will be balanced and the singer will be able to stand on tiptoe, on one leg, or walk away without radically changing the posture.

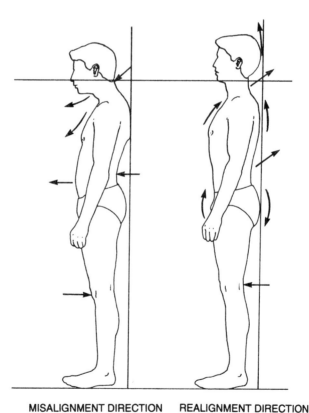

MISALIGNMENT DIRECTION   REALIGNMENT DIRECTION

Figure 11.3 Directions of postural realignment. (a) Poor posture, side view; (b) re-aligned, good posture, side view.

11.2.3. Checklist of Good Posture for Singing

The following points will ensure good posture for singing:

- head balanced comfortably at the top of the spine,
- back of the neck lengthened and the front loosened,
- jaw loose and released, and the chin free from any tendency to jut forward,
- the spine feeling long and wide
- back expanded 'open' with maximum space between shoulder blades,
- shoulders released down, and widened,
- chest comfortably raised and expanded,
- upper abdomen loose with the lower abdomen moving gently in and up to maintain the position of the pelvis, − (it is important that the pelvis not be in an exaggerated tucked position)
- knees unlocked and free,
- body weight distributed evenly on both the soles and heels of the feet,
- body weight balanced from front to back and from side to side.

From this poised, balanced, position the singer is ready to begin the cycle of activities that is responsible for creating and sustaining the singing voice. That cycle begins with the breath.

11.3 BREATHING

In the world of singing pedagogy, breathing and breath management are the subjects of much dispute, and a great deal of creative imagination has gone into methods proposed by various pedagogic schools. There is more than one way that breath can be generated by the respiratory system to create and sustain a given pitch [9].

11.3.1 Breathing and the Singer

When one moves from quiet breathing for conversational speech to the demands of singing, different physical and acoustical factors must be considered. The first of these concerns the implications of the larger lung volumes that are necessary to sustain steady musical phrases of average length. To understand this we must first review some of the facts relating to normal respiration and then compare them with the requirements of singing.

 If a normal man took in a full inhalation he would have in his lungs a total volume of between 6 and 7 liters. If he then exhaled as much air as he could, between 1.5 and 2 liters would still remain in his lungs. This difference of approximately 5 liters between the total lung capacity (TLC) of 7 liters and the residual volume (RV) of 2 liters is referred to as the vital capacity (VC).

 The full range of lung capacity is not often called into use, in fact the normal tidal volume used is really quite small. We breathe by means of a balanced mechanical system that contains both inhalatory and exhalatory forces acting as natural antagonists to each other. During quiet activity, or 'rest-breathing' these forces are constantly attempting to restore a state of equilibrium, as the respiratory pump alternates from predominantly exhalation to predominantly inhalation activity. Inhalation is a result of active muscle contractions expanding the lung volume, whilst exhalation is relatively passive, relying principally upon the elastic recoil in the ribs and lungs and the relaxation of the diaphragm to return to the functional residual capacity (FRC). The change in lung volume during quiet breathing is approximately 0.5 liters, in the range between 35% and 50% of the vital capacity. Figure 11.4 shows the relationship of these factors in diagrammatic form.

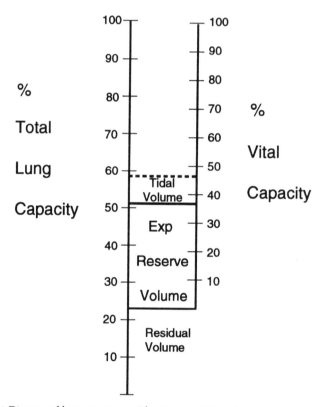

Figure 11.4 Diagram of lung capacities. (After Proctor [11], with permission.)

In singing and theatrical speech, the lung volume requirements change dramatically. During these activities, lung volumes range from 100% to 5% of vital capacity. Control of pressure and airflow rates over this volume range is more difficult because the positive and negative elastic recoil forces of the lung tissue, thorax, and abdomen have much greater values and influence the patterns of active forces applied to the respiratory system.

Proctor shows that after a maximum inhalation to TLC the passive elastic expiratory force of the lungs is approximately 20 cm H_2O, and that of the rib cage 10 cm H_2O [11]. This means that if uncontrolled, these two elastic forces alone can deliver a pressure of 30 cm H_2O at the onset of the expiratory cycle. This becomes of major technical significance to the singer when it is realized that only very loud singing requires this pressure. Most singing requires pressures in the range 5–20 cm H_2O and so it is clear that, without control, the system is applying excess pressure against the closed vocal folds (Figure 11.5). Whatever techniques singers choose to adopt, they must, to be safe and effective, control this elastic recoil and its attendant pressure levels, and present air to the larynx at a pressure appropriate for the desired pitch and loudness ('dynamic') level.

The solid line in Figure 11.5 represents the summation of the passive recoil forces generated by the rib cage and lungs. If the singer were to begin a vocal tone at a *pp* dynamic after a full breath he or she would, at this moment of onset, have to cope with an overpressure of approximately 25 cm H_2O, and this overpressure would continue to need controlling until the lung capacity was reduced to 55% of vital capacity. After this point a continuing tone would need expiratory effort to supply an adequate air pressure to the larynx. If however the starting dynamic had been at the *mf* requiring a 20 cm H_2O pressure level to sustain it, the overpressure would only exist down to approximately 86% of vital capacity after which the expiratory forces would need to assist.

With the constant changes of pitch and dynamic, and the ever-varying lung capacities that exist while the singer is in action, it can be clearly seen that the method of respiratory control that the singer adopts must be one of great flexibility and that any kind of forceful rigidities would render the necessary subtle actions impossible.

There is a common tendency among singers to give a deliberate inward kick with the abdominal musculature either at the onset of tone, or as an aid to upward pitch change. The effect of this action is to drive the diaphragm upward against the base of the lungs and so significantly increase the pressure of the contained air. If not carefully controlled, this action will destroy the essential balance between the desired subglottic pressure and pitch-making as well as the vocal fold adduction activities of the larynx.

Sundberg [13] indicates that a combination of the elastic recoil, muscle-driven rib descent, and diaphragm ascent, can generate subglottic pressures in excess of 150 cm H_2O. This means that the respiratory system is capable of delivering pressures that are five times greater than needed for most loud singing and almost eight times that required for an average vocal tone.

11.3.2 Techniques for the Control of Breathing

Breath control techniques for singing must create a balance between the pressure potential of the forces of exhalation and the desired subglottic pressure. It must be a very flexible arrangement that constantly changes with varying pitch and dynamic requirements, and with lung volume. There is evidence to suggest that muscles of inhalation are recruited as the natural antagonist to the exhalatory forces during

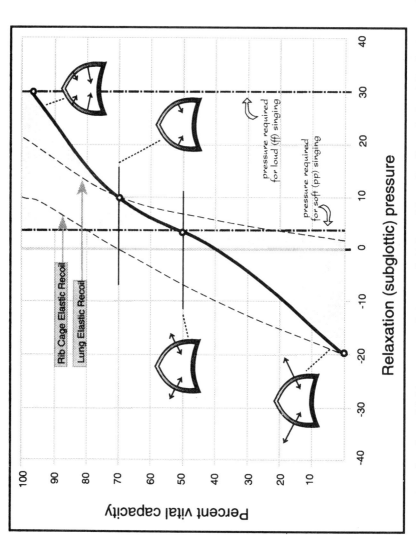

Figure 11.5 Pressures against closed vocal folds owing to elastic recoil. (Adapted from Sundberg [13] and Zemlin [16], with permission.)

phonation. The external intercostals and diaphragm may be most involved in creating the necessary balance of forces.

Watson and Hixon [15] found, during their study of classical singers, that there was a major discrepancy between the way their subjects thought they breathed and their observed patterns. Some singers can easily become tense and awkward if they try to think mechanically. However the process of inhalation for a singer must become more conscious than that of nonsingers, so that a full, relaxed breath is taken without extraneous tension.

Breathing in supine position

For many singers the easiest way to gain a sense of the breathing apparatus is to lie flat on the back, with a book supporting the head, legs bent with knees pointing upwards, and breathing slowly and comfortably through mouth and nose together (Figure 11.6). In this position, where the alignment of the spine and the position of the thorax is aided by the support of the floor, they will experience, on inhalation, expansion at the belt line and in the lower ribs. On exhalation they will feel the initiative taken by the muscles of the epigastric umbilical region of the abdomen to direct the outflow of the air. They will also note that there is little or no rise and fall of the upper chest during the breathing cycle.

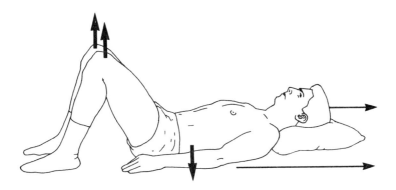

LYING SUPINE: LENGTHENING

Figure 11.6 Body in supine position, for breathing exercise.

Exercise

At a moderate tempo, breathe in for 5 counts, suspend the action for 5 counts, and then exhale for 5 counts. A complete and unforced expansion of the ribs and upper abdomen should be felt during the inhalation phase. The zone of maximum activity will be observed to be between the bottom of the sternum and the navel, and to extend all round the body to include the sides and the back. The lips should remain parted during the suspension phase, and there should be no feeling of the breath being held rigidly. The position of the ribs and upper abdomen should be comfortably retained. During exhalation the position of the sternum and the rib cage should be maintained as long as possible and only allowed to fall if necessary at the very end of the breath supply. The number of counts for each phase of the exercise can be increased steadily with growing efficiency up to a count of 10.

Variations can be made in the count patterns to develop the idea of the shorter inhalations and longer exhalations that musical compositions demand. Quicker inspiration and shorter suspension phases followed by a longer exhalation phase brings the sequence closer to the requirements of normal singing. Additional exercises can be introduced, sustaining for as long as comfortably possible the sibilant /s/ or the fricative /f/.

Breathing in standing position

The sensations and movement patterns that were experienced in the supine position should be retained as much as possible when the singer moves into standing position. There obviously will be some physical implications due to gravitational down-drag, but the body alignment should be similar, and most of the feelings learned in the supine position can be transferred to this upright position.

Exercise
Raise the arms above the head, bringing the sternum and ribs into a moderately high position. Allow the arms to fall back to the sides while the rib/sternum position is retained. The sternum should not be too high: this can be checked by seeing if it can be pushed even higher. From this comfortably high position it should be possible to breathe in and out easily without any rise or fall of the upper chest position. The previous exercises should then be experienced in this new upright position.

Exhalation phase of the breath cycle

The exhalation phase of the breath cycle is best considered in relation to phonation. It is at this point that most of the discord in singing pedagogy occurs because of the need to develop a technique for controlling elastic recoil, air flow, and subglottic pressures. The various schools of pedagogy instruct singers to push out with the stomach muscles, to keep the ribs expanded, to 'support', to pull the belly in, and even contract the muscles in their buttocks, all in the cause of achieving the desired control. A great deal of damage is done by this pushing and straining, in fact, more vocal problems are caused by forceful exhalation than by using the voice with no 'support' at all.

11.3.3 Summary of Breathing for Singing

It is a natural feature of the singing instrument that when a balance between the inhalatory and exhalatory forces has been established, the instrument can regulate the air flow rates and pressure values in direct response to the mental demands for pitch and dynamic. It is the singer's responsiblity to establish and maintain a physical environment wherein the subtle aerodynamic changes can take place.

Meribeth Bunch aptly sums up the breath action as follows, 'Support of tone is dependent upon maintenance of subglottic pressure. This is done by maintaining the inspiratory position of the rib cage for as long as possible while contracting the abdominal muscles and gradually relaxing the diaphragm. The inspiratory position of the rib cage implies a comfortably high (but not fixed or rigid) chest position so that there is no interference with the vibratory mechanism and no counteraction of expiratory effort. Maintenance of the inspiratory position ensures that at the onset of sound the inspiratory muscles remain in action, checking the elastic recoil of the lungs and rib cage' [5].

The following are some general principles for good breath management.

- Breathing for singing is dynamic, physical and muscular, rather than passive and uninvolved. It involves muscular antagonism.
- The singer needs an accurate concept of what takes place in the body during the process of breathing in and out. Although many of the same muscles are involved, it is different from weight lifting, vomiting, childbirth, and excretory functions.
- Strength and air capacity are of very little importance: coordination, skill, and experience are the main requirements. The action of the breathing mechanism should be so flexible that it will allow a new breath to be taken whenever the musical score presents an opportunity.
- Singers should not try to inhibit the flow of breath in singing phrases, rather they should allow the breath to move at all times. Let the voice 'call upon' the breath.
- Singers should not let the head position be affected by the attack or the release of the note.
- Singers should not push or aggressively attempt to 'support' the sound.

11.4 ONSET AND RELEASE OF VOCAL TONE

11.4.1 Onset

The most critical moment in the act of singing is the onset of the vocal tone. The term 'onset' is used in preference to the more frequently used term 'attack' as the latter is too suggestive of the clumsy and aggressive action that is at the root of so many singers' vocal problems. At this moment, the total singing instrument must be coordinated and balanced, and finely tuned to the desired pitch, vowel, and tonal quality. In the midst of such a complex operation the potential for imbalances and problems is great.

Sequence of events at tonal onset

At the end of a full inhalation the breath pressure in the lungs is equal to that of the surrounding atmosphere. The adductor muscles of the larynx move the vocal folds from their open inspiratory position, to a position where they meet at the midline and close the airway. Also at this time they are adjusted in length and tension to enable them to vibrate at the desired fundamental frequency. Once the airway is closed by the vocal folds the pressure can be adjusted to meet the pressure requirements of the desired pitch and dynamics. When this is established vocal fold vibrations can be initiated.

There are three kinds of onset that one observes in singing: the **soft** onset; the **hard** onset; and the **balanced** onset. One of these yields good results, another is inefficient, and the third is unhealthy. They are determined by the positioning and tension of the vocal folds within the above mentioned sequence.

Soft onset

In the soft onset, the sequence of events is slightly rearranged, in that there is a flow of breath that precedes the closure of the glottis producing an aspirate /h/ sound. The effect of this is to leave the glottis without firm closure. Visual observation often reveals an opening in the posterior glottis. The tonal effect is that of a soft, breathy, whispery quality, lacking both vibrancy and dynamic potential. This type of onset may represent chronic misuse of the laryngeal mechanism, described in Chapter 2 as the laryngeal isometric.

Hard onset

This is an action that is deserving of the word 'attack'. It is produced when the vocal folds are strongly adducted before phonation. The exaggerated adduction and medial compression forces result in high laryngeal resistance, thus demanding higher subglottic breath pressure to initiate phonation. The resulting glottic plosive is an audible unmusical preface to the sung tone. This kind of onset places considerable stress on the mechanism and carries potential for vocal fold damage. A similar chronic misuse may be noted in the speaking voice as well.

Balanced onset

The desirable, balanced onset occupies a position between these two extremes, and it produces a vibrant, full, resonant tone which has a distinct beginning and is free of any preliminary breathiness or launching bump. W.J. Henderson, the American critic and singing expert, who wrote on singing for the *New York Sun* and the *New York Times* from the mid 1880s to 1937 regarded the great soprano Nelli Melba as having the ideal vocal onset. At the time of her death in 1931, he wrote in the *New York Times*, 'The Melba attack was little short of marvelous. The term attack is not a good one. Melba indeed had no attack; she opened her mouth and a tone was in existence. It began without ictus, when she wished it to, and without betrayal of breathing. It simply was there. When she wished to make a bold attack, as in the trio of the last scene of "Faust," she made it with the clear silvery stroke of a bell' [8].

In the balanced onset the breathing mechanism stays in the expanded 'suspension' position at the moment of onset, and there is no inward movement of the umbilical epigastric region to destroy the balance between the vocal fold tension and the subglottic air pressure which has been established under the mental demand for pitch and dynamic. The result is a clean onset of sound which the singer often achieves by imagining a small aspirate /h/ before the sound but not allowing it to be audible, and by eliminating any sense of breath expulsion. It is important to remember that it is the manner of onset that determines the vocal sound that must follow, and the quality, intonation, carrying power, ease, and flexibility of the tone in the ensuing vocal phrase is determined in this moment.

11.4.2 Release

If the onset is the most critical moment in singing, then how the singer ends the tone – the release, follows a very close second in importance. The release at the end of a tone should be crisp and clean, with the glottis returning to the fully abducted position of deep inhalation. In other words, the release of the tone triggers a renewal of the breath, which in turn begins a new onset cycle of vocal tone. As was the case with the onset action, there are two undesirable forms of the release in addition to the ideal clean, crisp action. Again it is possible to have a 'hard' and a 'soft' version of the activity.

A 'hard' grunt-like release would cause the muscles to retain tension and prevent the vocal folds from returning to the fully abducted deep breathing position, thus delaying breath recovery, and efficient re-adduction. In the more common 'soft' release the muscle action is released slowly and the opening action is delayed, again slowing down the breath renewal action. This is further compounded by the fact that the sloppy, soft, release is usually accompanied by a collapse of the breathing mechanism and quite visible changes of posture are necessary in the attempts to renew the breath.

Exercises for the onset of tone were a feature of the training manuals of the early singing schools. These consisted of vocalises using sustained or staccato repeated notes on single or varying pitches which enabled repeated practice of the cycle of onset and release. The ideas that were stressed in these exercises were: clean onset, crisp release, and immediate breath renewal at the cessation of sound. The exercise sequence therefore conditions the muscles responsible for vocal fold approximation and glottic flexibility, and encourages quick, silent breath renewal.

11.5 RESONANCE

For singing, as for speaking, the sound that the vocal instrument produces is a direct product of the user's tonal imagination exercised within the limits of a naturally endowed physical framework. Speech precedes singing, and with some exceptions, a fine singing voice will be signalled by a fine speaking voice. The size of the voice, its ruggedness, and its resonance potential are basic features of the natural gift, but every singer can maximize the resonance and color of the voice. Beauty of tone is not only a feature of natural gift, it is the result of balanced resonance with unforced, comfortable tone. Unfortunately, many problems arise from the singer's desire to maximize the power and carrying capacity of the voice at the expense of natural free resonance and other, more subtle features.

What must be understood about the singing voice is that it is an instrument that can, for our purposes, be considered to house two vibrating systems: the vocal folds; and the air contained in the vocal tract above the larynx. Each of these is adjustable; the former by the actions of their intrinsic musculature in response to the demands for pitch, and the latter by adjustments in the size and configuration of the oral and pharyngeal spaces which use the tongue, palate, jaw, and lips to respond to demands for vowel and tonal texture or quality. What is essential for the best quality of sound is that these two systems vibrate in sympathy with each other. Failure to find this sympathetic relationship will be revealed in tones that are lacking in vibrancy, beauty, clarity, and freedom.

To produce a singing tone of acceptable aesthetic quality, the resonance system of the voice selects for enhancement those harmonics from the laryngeal signal that are sympathetic with the overtone series of the desired sung pitch. Only a resonance system that is sympathetically tuned to the frequency of the vibrator can successfully carry out these processes of selection and enhancement. An unsympathetic resonator would be inclined to either enhance the wrong things, or be limited in the extent to which it could enhance the harmonics of the sung pitch. The tonal result would be either ugly, weak, or both. For the singer the feeling would be one of effort, discomfort, and lack of freedom.

11.5.1 Tonal Concept as a Control Factor

The major control factor in bringing about this sympathetic relationship between the voice source vibrator and that of the resonance system is the singer's concept of vocal tone. This tonal model is a mental concept based on imagery and experience, and ranks in importance with tonal onset and release. This is the device the brain uses to trigger major muscular adjustments in the resonatory system, and its model must be appropriate to the natural physical parameters of the instrument as well as the aesthetic objectives of the vocal tone.

There are many ways in which this crucial technical requirement can go astray, and in almost every case the cause has its genesis in the singer's desire to create a tonal sound that is not appropriate to his or her natural instrument. A common case is a desire to produce a bigger sound than one can accommodate. The tonal model is also often distorted by singers who want to make their voices sound like their favorite artists regardless of the differences in age and physical endowment. Among opera singers, the dramatic and tessitura demands of an unsuitable role cause the singer to seek an inappropriate tone. Among pop singers it is the urge to copy, for obvious monetary reasons, the sound of those who are commercially successful, again regardless of physical endowment or racial background.

The model that the singer creates must contain within it several factors all of which must be appropriate to the natural endowment of the singer in question, including the size, colour, emotional quality, and dramatic intent of the tone; plus a precise definition of vowel form and pitch.

Any miscalculation in the concept of these elements can have serious implications for the freedom and dynamics of the vocal instrument. For example, attempts to sing too big a tonal sound invariably lead to generation of an excessive driving pressure, and defensive hypervalving in the larynx. This aggressive action of the breath and the consequent laryngeal reaction is highly fatiguing for the larynx, and leads to a tonal sound that is shouty and usually faulty in pitch. Attempts to create an inappropriately dramatic sound have some of the problems of the previous fault pattern plus a tendency to overexaggerate the lower harmonics in the spectrum, making the tonal sound heavy, with poor pitch and vowel definition.

On the other hand many singers, in their attempts to sing quietly, allow the sound to lose its vibrancy, with weak adduction of the vocal folds and inadequate subglottic pressure, leading to a breathy tone and erratic intonation.

11.5.2 An Approach to Vocal Freedom and Tonal Modelling

Perhaps the most constructive approach is to assume that the voice will respond freely to the appropriate mental tonal model if muscle tensions in the throat, jaw, and tongue do not interfere with the natural, effective coordination of the breath and the larynx. The release of these tensions, should they exist, is directed by the singing teacher in a number of ways.

- The vowels should be formed with a loose jaw and a forward, relaxed tongue, allowing the resonance of the voice to grow as coordination with the breath increases.
- Onsets should be properly coordinated, with no breathiness nor with an exaggerated glottic attack. Staccato exercises have traditionally been used for this, as have long legato phrases for 'seating' the vowel in the breath.
- Pitch and articulation should be flexible. When the voice is flexible, it is likely that there is good coordination and little unnecessary tension. Exercises in scales, arpeggios and quick sequential patterns have traditionally helped singers become skillful and relaxed.
- Relaxed but refined speech should be practiced and it should have technical similarities to singing.

Strategies for developing good resonance include the following.

- Development of appropriate tonal models: let the singer hear the accomplishments of other similar voices with good techniques.
- Use of a variety of environments for singing, and alterations of acoustic feedback of the singer's own voice, by covering the ears, making a megaphone of the hands, etc.
- Use of tape-recorders to help in learning that the sounds which are most resonant to the listener are probably not those most resonant to the singer.

11.6 IMAGERY IN VOCAL PEDAGOGY

In the world of singing pedagogy, extensive use is made of mental imagery to try and gain technical control over the instrument, and some of these images can be considered as another aspect of modelling, as discussed above. Words such as 'focus' and 'placement', 'head voice' and 'chest voice' all have the effect of influencing the relationship between the vibratory and the resonatory systems of the voice. Although there may be some value to these images, in general they do not provide precise directives and as a result they are the source of much confusion and vocal abuse. Efforts to 'place the voice in the mask', in the name of resonance and placement, are often ineffective and usually result in an ugly, pinched tone, and a host of other problems.

While there is potential for problems to develop from the use of ill-defined or vague imagery it must also be recognized that it is by these means that we gain access to the control of the voice. The previous discussion on tonal modelling and its influence upon pitch, dynamics, and resonance, makes that point.

The problem relates to those images that are inspired by the physical sensations that the singer experiences during the act of singing. 'Focus', 'placement', 'forward sounds', 'backward sounds', 'head voice', 'chest voice', are all products of the very real sensory experiences of the singer in action. But many of the sensory impressions that a singer receives convey either vague or inaccurate information about the location or the specifics of the events taking place.

11.6.1 Tonal Placement

A good example of this sensory experience is that of the singer who makes a ringing tonal sound having a good, strong singer's formant in the 2800–3500 Hz range. He or she will often experience strong sympathetic vibrations in the sinus regions. What the singer is actually experiencing is a strong resonance response from those cavities whose own natural frequencies happen to coincide with those of the singer's formant. To the singer however, it feels as though the sound is securely placed 'forward' and 'in the mask', and it is hard to diminish the conviction that this secure feeling is merely a secondary factor and not the primary cause of such a desired and praised vocal tone. This could be nothing more than a harmless self-deception if it were not for the fact that many schools of voice pedagogy devote time and effort to 'place' the vocal tone into particular sinus regions, sometimes, sadly, with not too much regard for what may be going on in the instrument to achieve this result. There are, in fact, several possible ways to achieve this sense of 'forward placement', some of which can have a negative effect on the singing voice. The sensation of 'forward placement' that comes as a result of a well-produced vocal tone is 'real' to the singer. What must be recognized is that the primary generator of these sensations is located elsewhere in the resonance system, in particular the laryngeal cavity.

11.6.2 Registers and Range

Similar confusion is created by the sympathetic sensations experienced in the cavities of the skull in the higher pitch range, and the chest cavity in the lower pitch range, which gives rise to the images of 'head' and 'chest' voice. These sensory impressions have contributed significantly to the confusion in terminology and understanding of vocal registers, and it is hard to convince some singers that these sensations contribute nothing to the tonal quality of the sound product that the audience experiences.

11.6.3 Breath Support

The concept of 'breath support' also appears to be born out of the singer's sensations of the activity in the lower thoracic and upper abdominal region. In the balanced breath-suspension action described earlier, a 'support-like' sensation is associated with the natural antagonistic actions of the diaphragmatic, thoracic, and abdominal musculature, and the intensity of this relationship varies with the rise and fall of pitch and tonal dynamic. While this feeling of 'support' is a very real sensation to the singer, it is imperative that it be understood that this range of muscle activities is produced reflexively in response to the mental demands for pitch and dynamic. It must not be construed from these sensations that the way to control pitch or loudness is to deliberately push down on the diaphram, pull in on the abdomen, or create various deliberate contortions with the thoracic muscles.

11.6.4 Open Throat

The concept of an 'open throat' is another image that is much sought after by the singer and voice teacher. For the singer whose voice is working well there is a sensation of freedom, openness, and space in the oropharyngeal cavities. What the singer is responding to is in fact the absence of undesirable, constrictive tensions in the system, usually in the posterior part of the tongue, the pharynx, and within the larynx itself. To the singer the throat feels 'open', and this is desirable.

Many pedagogic notions are employed to try and remove potential obstructions and recreate this 'open-throated' posture on a regular basis; these include flattening the tongue, raising the soft palate, inflating the pharynx, and lowering the larynx to various levels. Often the yawn reflex is co-opted to assist in the cause. It is true that the yawn reflex, in the moment that it begins, causes a sense of release and a comfortable sense of easy increase in the size of the oropharyngeal cavity. If it could be made to stop there all would be well and the image of a 'gentle yawn' would have considerable pedagogic value. Unfortunately this reflex is difficult to control and continues to the next stage of its pattern which is a major distention of the whole oropharyngeal space, and tongue retraction. All this new-found 'yawny' space gives singers a feeling of 'openness' of the throat, but all they really have is a retracted tongue, rigidity in the palate, an overly depressed larynx, and a distended pharynx. It may feel 'open', but in such an environment the essential singing activities of articulation and the constant readjustment of the resonance cavity coupling is rendered virtually impossible. This begs the question: What is the singer's 'open throat'? The answer is: There is no such entity in the way we would like to imagine it.

11.6.5 Problems of Imagery

The problem with the use of imagery is that it is often inaccurate as a description of events, and is usually sufficiently vague as to allow almost infinite interpretation. In 1931 Dr G.O. Russell published in his book *Speech and Voice* some radiographic images of famous singers that were taken during the production of the vowel sounds /i/, /ɑ/, and /u/ [12]. These were mid-sagittal views of the head showing the position of the tongue, palate, epiglottis, and the general configuration of the resonance tract. In 1959 he was able to indentify some of these images as being of the great tenor Enrico Caruso, who, it appears, was so dismayed upon seeing them that he refused to allow his name to be associated with them. What concerned him was the fact that they did not bear out his own sensory perceptions: the /ɑ/ and /u/ vowels with their natural constriction between the back of the tongue and the back wall of the throat belied his sensory feeling of an 'open throat', and the complete closure of his palate did not show 'the resonance of the nasal passages being properly utilized'. As Berton Coffin in *Overtones of Bel Canto* comments, 'He could not accept the truth of the matter – fancy being stronger than fact' [6].

Coffin also suggests by way of explanation that the so-called huge space of the /ɑ/ vowel in the throat is a fiction, and that, because of the small opening between the epiglottis and the back wall of the throat, a zone of high pressure is felt in this area which is probably what gives the singer a feeling of space.

11.6.6 Images as a Teaching Tool

The teacher can never be sure that the imagery and terminology that is used will trigger in the student the same sensations that it does in the teacher. It is important therefore that the teacher and the singer, working together, develop a vocal technique in which the sensations experienced by the singer are related to the actual desired physiological and acoustical events. If this can be done then the sensations that singers feel so strongly, can become their confirmation of the correctness of their vocal actions. They can apply what ever imagery they like to these experiences. The images can then become the means that singers use to keep in contact with their instrument in the midst of the complexities and distractions of vocal performance.

If singers and voice teachers could develop a clearer understanding of cause and effect in vocal activity, and an exact and direct technical language to communicate that understanding, a great deal could be done to clear away the confusion that bedevils the field of voice pedagogy.

11.7 REGISTERS AND RANGE

Vocal registers and the development of the singer's working range are so bound together that a lack of mechanical understanding and technical knowledge of the former can lead to serious limitations of access and usage of the latter.

A review of available literature will quickly show that this is one of the areas of vocal technique about which there is much confusion and disagreement. The modern-day singer is confronted with a set of opinions regarding registers that range from the existence of no registers at all to the possibility of seven, the prize for popularity going to the idea of two for males and three for females. It is imperative to the development and vocal survival of singers that they make some effort to come to an understanding of this phenomenon and find a practical way to deal with it in their every day vocal activities. To fail to do so can lead to severe limitations in range and tonal quality.

Even after singers arrive at some satisfactory concept of the number of registers existing in their voices, they are still confronted with the problem of what to call them.

11.7.1 Register Terminology

There has developed over time a terminology that, rather than clarifying the issue, has added to the confusion. Maybe the heart of the problem stems from attempts throughout much of the history of singing to explain and label the phenomenon of vocal registers from the point of view of the singer's sensations of physical and resonance phenomena. The understanding and terminology that stems from this process does little to help the singer come to terms with the physiological events that are actually taking place. Let us consider the singers' sensory experiences as they ascend through their vocal ranges. As one progresses from the bottom to the top of the pitch range, one experiences, at certain points in the progression, changes in sensory perception that gives one the impression that physical and resonance adjustments are taking place. The lower pitches seem to excite strong vibrations in the chest, while on the middle pitches the sensation moves up to the hard palate and into the oropharyngeal cavity. In the higher pitches it feels as though the vibrations are taking place higher in the head. The series of notes in each of these groups also have a similar tonal timbre (quality), and for each group there is a sense of a specific adjustment of the breathing mechanism.

Because of these powerful subjective experiences, there appeared quite early in the history of singing an attempt to use the singer's sensations to describe the actual physical events. Hence we had 'chest voice', 'head' or 'falsetto' voice, and later on, 'middle voice'. This latter was sometimes subdivided into 'upper middle' and 'lower middle' to represent those tones that felt as though they still retained an affinity to the 'head' or the 'chest' voice. There was also a gender difference in this early assessment, female voices being assigned three registers, 'chest', 'middle', and 'head', and male voices assigned two, 'chest', and 'falsetto'.

The term 'falsetto' has also had a confusing history of its own. On the one hand it was used to represent the upper register of the male voice, though some believe the earlier schools of singing employed this term to refer to a more vibrant upper register and not the quasi-feminine sounds that the male voice is capable of making. On the other hand the great and influential voice teacher Manuel Garcia really muddied the waters when he used this term to represent the 'middle' register, saying that it constituted a particular register that differed from both the 'head' and the 'chest' register, and was located between them [7]. To the 20th century singer, 'falsetto' has come to represent that quasi-feminine sound that the male voice is capable of producing in the upper part of the vocal range.

What terminology should we use? Voice scientists have suggested that since there is so much confusion, and as the old labels don't accurately describe what is occurring mechanically in the larynx, we should adopt the terms applied to speaking voice registers as defined by the vibratory patterns of the vocal folds. Using the speaking register terms, 'modal' would incorporate 'chest' voice, and 'loft' or 'falsetto' might replace 'head' register. This terminology may simplify descriptions but does not really help singers relate to the precise sensations and timbral differences they experience, so by itself is not likely to gain popular useage among the singing fraternity. A more valuable approach would combine mechanical physiological, acoustic and sensory aspects of registers.

11.7.2 Current Understanding About Registers

One of the best, and most comprehensive definitions of singing registers is by Nadoleczeny and Zimmerman [10] and dates back to 1937:

> A register within the human vocal scale is a series of sounds of equal quality. The musical ear distinguishes them from another series of sounds also of equal quality. The limits of each series are marked by 'points' of passage sometimes called 'lifts'. The timbre of each series, or register, is the result of a constant rapport of harmony. To the male singer the primary register change at the upper part of the scale gives a certain vibrating sensation perceptible to the head. To the female the primary register change at the lower part of the scale gives a certain vibratory sensation in the chest. Each area of identical quality depends upon the adjustment of the resonating cavities. Registers are produced by a mechanism that functions in the production of sound. The principal characteristic of this mechanism is the manner in which a particular vibration is coupled with the supraglottic and the infraglottic resonators.

So where does all this leave would-be singers with their desire to obey both the mechanical and aesthetic rules as they progress up and down the scale? From the outset it is important to state that at this point in time, while the findings of the voice scientists have enabled us to understand a great deal about the workings of the laryngeal and resonance mechanisms, unknowns still exist regarding singing registers. There is, however, sufficient knowledge to plot a strategy and a pedagogic approach to the matter of vocal registers. In a practical approach there would appear to be a need to understand registers as both a resonance and a mechanical phenomenon and to acknowledge that the events coincide and interact.

11.7.3. Registers as a Mechanical Phenomenon

In order to establish a particular fundamental frequency it is necessary that the vocal folds assume a specific degree of tension and mass per area. Assuming the appropriate driving forces are adjusted to accommodate glottic resistance changes, f_0 rises as length (and thus ligament tension) increases and mass per area decreases, and f_0 falls as the ligament tension relaxes and mass per area increases. The cricothyroid muscles are those principally responsible for adjusting length, but the effective length change depends on antagonistic anchoring forces of the crico-arytenoid muscles. The thyroarytenoid muscles may contract to adjust tension or mass per area of the folds.

Physiologically, we have on a scalar ascent a gradual increase in vocal fold tension and a diminishing of vocal fold mass per area, which is achieved by the different laryngeal muscle groups taking varying degrees of responsibility as the pitch rises. The ideal, to comply with the aesthetics of most western music, is that this shifting of responsibility be carried out as smoothly and as unobtrusively as possible.

11.7.4 Model of Vocal Registers

Despite differences of opinion there is a model of registration events that makes accommodation for the differing voice categories and even accommodates important subdivisions within those categories.

It will be noticed in Figure 11.7 that, in this model, each register has its own range of notes, and although the diagram suggests that each register ends at a precise point there is in fact usually a zone of overlap between the ending point of one register and the beginning point of the one above. In this area the singer can choose to sing the required notes in either register, always bearing in mind that the notes at the top of a register demand a higher work load from the muscles than the bottom notes of the register above.

11.7.5 Useful Analogy of Register Mechanics

It has been suggested by Godfrey Arnold that the mechanical events of the ascending and descending vocal scale are somewhat like the events of the gear-shifts in a car as it increases and decreases speed. [3] Though this analogy may not quite represent the smooth and graduated transitions that singing desires, we can use it to demonstrate the issue of locus of control for register transitions. For the automobile, when the gear shift is primarily in the hands of the driver (standard transmission), he or she has a choice of either driving in a low gear at high r.p.m. or using fewer engine revolutions in a higher gear. Some drivers may not appreciate the principles of efficient use of the mechanism, so may continue to accelerate without bothering to change gear at all, in other words they may choose to let the r.p.m. go on increasing as the car gathers speed. This misuse can lead to an overheated engine and mechanical breakdown. A similar stress on the mechanism arises if gear changing is done clumsily, or mistimed, all of which is made apparant by the noise of grinding gears or the kangaroo-like progression of the car as it goes down the road. In all these cases the effect on the car's gearbox and engine will be most unhealthy and an early visit to the mechanic a certainty.

A similar set of possibilities confronts the singer. It is possible that, because of the singer's tonal imagery, mechanical ineptitude, or the demands of certain musical styles,

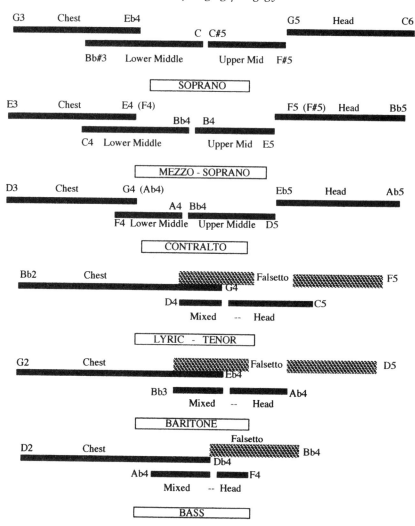

Figure 11.7 Diagram of traditional models of register location and points of register transition.

that the appropriate mechanical adjustments that facilitate pitch changes are delayed or can not take place at all. The most potentially harmful of these events are those that force a lower register adjustment higher than is appropriate, causing muscles to assume a hypertonic state. In other words the engine is wilfully driven at high r.p.m. values.

The most commonly seen examples of this abuse are attempts to overextend the 'chest' register with laryngeal hypervalving and aggressive use of the breathing mechanism. While the choice of the lower register can be made for occasional artistic effect (loud tones at the upper border of a register will nearly always continue to engage the lower mechanism, whereas piano tones are likely to adopt the next higher registration), a working rule of thumb would be: if in doubt, switch to the upper registration on the ascending scale.

In the world of 'pop' music and musical theatre, the demand that all singers, regardless of their natural endowment, produce a predetermined type of vocal tone throughout their working range, frequently leads to a refusal to allow the natural register adjustments to take place, often with negative results both musically and for the singers' health.

11.7.6 Vocal Registers as a Resonance Phenomenon

In Chapter 10 the acoustical characteristics of the harmonic spectrum generated by the vocal folds and the formant structures of the vocal tract transfer function are discussed. We need to review these phenomena since they may account for much of the sensory perception that a singer experiences of the register events. It is by the choice and manipulation of the resonance characteristics that the singer can influence and enhance the pitch progression, and most pedagogical techniques dealing with registration are based on this assumption. This therefore requires an understanding of the interaction of harmonics and vowel formants.

Harmonics

The vibratory action of the vocal folds produces a complex signal that delivers into the resonance tract a series of harmonics that are mathematically predictable relative to the f_0 of the sung tone. The first harmonic is always one octave above the fundamental (two times the f_0); the second, another octave above (three times the f_0) Figure 11.8 shows the harmonic series assuming, for convenience, that a bass is singing a low C.

Because of the mathematical designation of harmonics in the voice source spectrum, the density of harmonics that the vocal tract responds to acoustically depends upon the sung fundamental. A bass voice, which operates at relatively low f_0 levels, can generate in the vocal tract a dense spectrum of harmonics, since multiplication of the lower f_0 will predict a greater number of harmonics within a given resonator's frequency range. A Soprano with her higher f_0 range cannot create so many harmonics for the same frequency range of a resonator. This simple voice source principle accounts for some of the basic differences in the tonal colours of the two voice categories. Luckily, the male and female vocal tracts are designed to enhance different parts of the harmonic frequency range. The larger male tract is particularly suited to resonate lower frequency harmonics, and the resonance capability of the smaller female tract provides potential power to higher frequency harmonics of the voice source spectrum.

Interaction of formants and harmonics

Formant frequencies depend upon the length and the shape of the vocal tract and the values will vary for the different voice categories and the size and shape of an individual's vocal tract.

The acoustical effect of the supraglottic cavity shapes is that each subpocket of space tends to be sympathetic to a specific narrow frequency range. Any harmonic whose

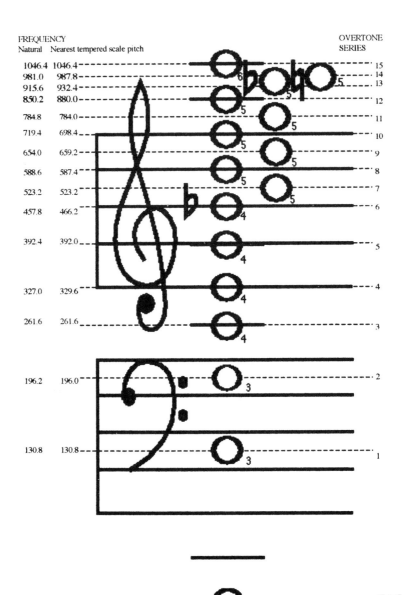

Figure 11.8 The harmonic sequence. (After Vennard [14], with permission.)

natural frequency coincides with those favored by the subpockets of the vowel-shaped resonatory tract will be reinforced. Other nonsympathetic harmonics would be dampened. Please refer to Chapter 10 to see how the harmonic spectrum is influenced by the vocal tract to adjust for various vowels.

Both the quality and the identification of a given vowel sound is determined by the presence, within its harmonic spectrum, of certain reinforced harmonics. The ear has been trained to recognize that certain vowels sounds are represented by the reinforcement of harmonics at specific frequencies.

Appelman [2] has provided us with average frequencies of the first three formant bands for the basic singing vowels in our language (Table 11.1). It is important to realize that these values mark the center of an allowable range and that some variation in the values will still enable vowel intelligibility.

Table 11.1 List of frequencies for the first three formants in the male and female voice

	Male				Female		
Phoneme	f_1	f_2	f_3	*Phoneme*	f_1	f_2	f_3
/i/	300	1950	2750	/i/	400	2250	3300
/I/	375	1810	2500	/I/	475	2125	3450
/e/	450	1800	2480	/e/	500	1900	3250
/ɛ/	530	1500	2500	/ɛ/	550	1750	3250
/æ/	620	1490	2250	/æ/	600	1650	3000
/a/	650	1200	2500	/a/	675	1555	3300
/ɔ/	610	1000	2600	/ɔ/	625	1240	3250
/o/	450	700	2500	/o/	500	1000	3000
/U/	400	720	2550	/U/	425	900	3375
/u/	350	640	2550	/u/	450	800	3250
/ɑ/	700	1200	2600	/ɑ/	700	1300	3250

(Data from Appelman [2].)

From Table 11.1 we can see that the first formants occur outside the normal working range of most male voice singing, the exception being the very top notes of the bass and baritone, and the 'head' register of the tenor.

In the female voice we see that the formant values are somewhat higher, and that the first formants occur in the pitch range occupied mostly by the 'middle' register of the voice.

To summarize, as the pitch ascends and descends it is necessary that there be changes in the specific harmonics that the formants choose to boost. These changes of harmonic selection are influenced not only by pitch variation, but also by changing vowel forms. In plotting the points of change in the harmonic formant relationship throughout all the vowel sounds and ranges of both the female and male voices, it is interesting to note that major changes do tend to take place consistently in certain zones of the voice, and there is a tendency for these formant harmonic changes to shadow the accepted registration change points of the traditional pedagogical schools.

For singers there is often an awareness of both physical change at strategic points in the upward progress of their scale, and also of the need to manipulate the tonal qualities and the vowel forms to assist in a smooth passage through these points of change. There is a possibility that these mechanical and acoustical events, often occurring on the same pitches, are an unrelated coincidence, but one that traditional schools have noticed and tried to resolve for centuries. Despite the apparent differences in pedagogical opinion on this matter, it is interesting to note that in the traditional pedagogies nearly all the suggested solutions to the supposed mechanical events of register changes result in an adjustment of the resonance factors and the formant harmonic relationship. These techniques recommend vowel modification, palatal adjustment, adding 'nasal' resonance, adjustment of laryngeal elevation, 'covering' the tone, keeping the tone 'focused', etc.

11.7.7 Range

The full range of the voice can be achieved by the skillful use of the different registers and the most productive attitude is to begin with the concept that there are no 'ceilings' or fixed boundaries, only points of transition. The knowledge of where these transition points are in each individual voice, combined with the singers' own sensory feedback, enable them to make the necessary adjustments with both safe and artistically satisfying results.

Singers should be careful not to allow the categorization of voices to become some kind of psychological barrier to the exploration of range and registers. While the repertoire that is traditionally assigned to specific voice categories presupposes a working range for that particular voice category, the quality and timbre of the voice also play a major part in the determination. Each singer will have his or her own naturally endowed pitch range and it is this personal exploration that must take place.

The prerequisite to working in range development should be the ability to sustain free and resonant vocal tones in that part of the singer's range that is most easily accessible. This zone is usually initially determined by the range of the modal register we use for free and natural speech activities (but not the low-pitched and monotone 'authority-figure' voice, nor speech in the glottic fry register). From this secure base the exploration and development of the range can begin. Simple patterns of scales and arpeggios, that take the voice progressively throughout its full range and through all registers, can be developed to accomplish this work of range development. It is important that the upper range be sung lightly at first, and higher notes should not necessarily imply an increase in volume and a sense of strain.

References

1. Alexander F.M. (1932) *The Use of the Self*, Methuen London.
2. Appelman D.R. (1967) *The Science of Vocal Pedagogy*, 1974, Reprint, Indiana University, Bloomington IN.

3. Arnold G (1969) Research potential in voice registers, in *vocal Registers in Singing* (ed. J.W. Large) Mouton, The Hague.
4. Barlow W (1973) *The Alexander Technique*, Healing Arts Rochester, VT.
5. Bunch M (1982) *Dynamics of the Singing Voice*, Springer New York, NY. Verlag
6. Coffin B (1980) *Overtones of Bel Canto*, Scarecrow, Metuchen, NJ.
7. Garcia M (1854;1855) Observations on human voice. *Proceedings of the Royal Society of London*, **7**, 399–410.
8. Henderson W.J. (1938) *The Art of Singing*, 1968 reprint, Book for Libraries, Freeport, NY.
9. Hixon T.J. (1987) *Respiratory Function in Speech and Song*, College-Hill, Boston, MA.
10. Nadoseczeny M ed Zimmerman R (1937) Catégories et régistres de la voix. *Revue Franççaise de Phoniatre*, January, 21–31.
11. Proctor D.F. (1980) *Breathing, Speech and Song*, Springer, New York, NY.
12. Russell G.O. (1931) *Speech and Voice*, MacMillan, New York, NY.
13. Sundberg J (1987) *The Science of the Singing Voice*, Northern Illinois University, Dekalb, IL.
14. Vennard W (1967) *Singing, the Mechanism and the Technic*, Carl Fischer, New York, NY.
15. Watson P.J. ed Hixon T.J. (1985) Respiratory kinematics in classical (opera) singers. *Journal of Speech and Hearing Research*, **28**, 104–22.
16. Zemlin W.R. (1988) *Speech and Hearing Science: Anatomy and Physiology* 3rd ed, Prentice-Hall, Englewood Cliffs, NJ.

Appendix A

Antireflux instructions

In some people, irritating acid stomach juices may leak out of the stomach and into the esophagus and throat. This causes irritation and muscle spasm in the throat. Some of the symptoms that people have from this include coughing, burning or soreness, throat clearing, excess mucus, bad taste and a sensation of a lump in the throat.

The following instructions are designed to help neutralize the stomach, reduce the production of acid and prevent acid from coming up the esophagus. You should use as many of these symptoms as needed to get relief. If these measures do not help, or if your symptoms get worse, you should let me know about it.

- Take an antacid in liquid form (Gelusil, Maalox, or others of your choice – Tums may be OK) 30–40 minutes after meals and at bedtime. If symptoms are severe, take antacids every one-and-a-half or two hours between meals.
- If you are overweight, you should lose weight.
- Diet restrictions help control symptoms. A bland diet divided into multiple, small feedings is recommended. You should avoid highly seasoned food, fats, citrus, tomato, onion, pepper, commercial potato chips and fried foods. Other things that promote reflux include chocolate, nuts, pastries, olives and vegetable oil. Each meal should include protein for stability (e.g., meat, fish, eggs, chicken, cottage cheese). Care should be taken to chew food properly.
- Alcohol, tobacco, and coffee are irritants to the esophagus and should be avoided. Alcohol and coffee also stimulate acid stomach secretions. Avoid all strongly flavoured candies, lozenges, gum, breath fresheners, etc.
- Do not eat for three or four hours before retiring.
- For night-time relief, sleep with the head of your bed elevated since symptoms are more likely to occur if you lie flat. The best way to achieve elevation is to place cinder blocks, wood, or bricks under the legs of the head of the bed. The desired elevation ranges from 4 to 8 inches (10–20 cm), with 6 inches (15 cm) a customary average. If this is not practical, sleep on two or three pillows or a foam wedge. Sometimes sleeping on the right side prevents distressing attacks.
- Clothing that fits tightly across the mid-section of the body should be avoided. Women should not wear a girdle. Men should not wear a belt, but should use suspenders (braces) instead. Use of 'abdominal supporting belts' should be prohibited.

- You should practice abdominal or diaphragmatic breathing when you are having symptoms. This means that you concentrate on pushing out the stomach with each breath instead of expanding the chest.
- Do not bend or stoop any more than is absolutely necessary. This includes activities such as gardening and exercises requiring lifting or bending.
- Maintaining a relaxed attitude in your activities helps to reduce symptoms.

Adapted from D.N. Olson, with permission.

Appendix B

Vocal rehabilitation exercises

B.1 VOCAL HYGIENE: HOW TO GET THE BEST MILEAGE FROM YOUR VOICE

Don't Abuse Your Voice

- Don't clear your throat or cough habitually.
    Instead: − yawn to relax your throat;
        − swallow slowly, drink some water;
        − hum: concentrate on vocal resonance sensations.
- Don't yell, cheer, or scream habitually.
    Instead: − use nonvocal sounds to attract attention: clap, whistle, ring a bell, blow a horn;
        − find nonvocal ways to train/discipline children and pets.
    Avoid prolonged talking over long distances and outside.
    Instead: − move closer, so you can be heard without yelling;
        − learn good vocal projection techniques.
- Avoid talking in noisy situations: over loud music, office equipment, noisy classrooms, or public places; in cars, buses, aeroplanes.
    Instead: − reduce background noise in your daily environment;
        − always face persons you are speaking with;
        − position yourself close to your listeners;
        − wait until students/audience are quiet and attentive;
        − find nonvocal ways to elicit attention.
- Don't try to address large audiences without proper amplification. You should be able to lecture at a comfortable loudness to be heard in any situation.
    Instead: − use a microphone for public speaking;
        − learn microphone technique.
- Don't sing beyond your comfortable range.
    Instead: − know your physical limits for pitch and loudness;
        − seek professional vocal training;
        − always use an adequate monitoring system to guide your voice use during performance;
        − never sing a high note that you can't sing quietly.

- Avoid vocally abusive nervous habits of public speaking: throat-clearing breath-holding speaking quickly, speaking on insufficient breath, speaking on low, monotone pitch, aggressive or low-pitched fillers: *um . . ., ah. . . .*
  Instead: – monitor and reduce vocal habits that detract from your presentation;
  – learn strategies for effective public speaking.
- Don't speak extensively during strenuous physical exercise.
  Instead: – avoid loud and aggressive vocal 'grunts';
  – after aerobic exercise, wait until your breathing system can accommodate optimal voice production.

Don't Misuse Your Voice

- Don't talk with a low-pitched monotone voice. Don't allow your vocal energy to drop so low that the sound becomes rough and gravelly ('glottic fry')
  Instead: – keep your voice powered by breath flow, so the tone carries, varies, and rings;
  – allow your vocal pitch to vary as you speak.
- Don't hold your breath as you're planning what to say. Avoid tense voice onsets ('glottic attacks').
  Instead: – keep your throat relaxed as you begin speaking;
  – use the breathing muscles and airflow to start speech phrases: the coordinated voice onset.
- Don't speak beyond a natural breath cycle: avoid squeezing out the last few words of a thought with insufficient breath power.
  Instead: – speak slowly, pausing often at natural phrase boundaries, so your body can breathe naturally.
- Don't tighten your upper chest, shoulders, neck, and throat to breathe in, or to push sound out.
  Instead: – allow your body to stay aligned and relaxed so breathing is natural;
  – allow your abdomen and rib cage to move freely.
- Don't clench your teeth, tense your jaw or tongue.
  Instead: – keep your upper and lower teeth separated;
  – let your jaw move freely during speech;
  – learn specific relaxation exercises.
- Avoid prolonged use of unconventional vocal sounds: whispering, growls, squeaks, imitating animal, or machine noises . . .
  Instead: – If you must talk when your voice is strained, use a soft, vocal tone instead of a loud, harsh whisper;
  – If you must produce special vocal effects for performance, make sure you are using a technique that minimizes muscle tension and vocal abuse,
- When you sing, don't force your voice to stay in a register beyond its comfortable pitch range. Especially, don't force your 'chest voice' too high; and don't force your 'head voice' high into falsetto range.
  Instead: allow vocal registers to change with pitch;

− consult your singing teacher to learn techniques for smooth register transitions.

Maintain a Healthy Lifestyle and a Healthy Environment

- Don't demand more of your voice than you would the rest of your body.
  Instead: − allow for several periods of voice rest throughout the day.
- Don't use your voice extensively or strenuously when you are sick, or when you feel tired.
  Instead: − rest your voice with your body: It's sick too!
- Don't use your voice when it feels strained.
  Instead: − Learn to be sensitive to the first signs of vocal fatigue: hoarseness, throat tension, dryness,
- Don't ignore prolonged symptoms of vocal strain, hoarseness, throat pain, fullness, heartburn, or allergies.
  Instead: − consult your doctor if you experience throat symptoms or voice change for more than 10 days.
- Don't expose your voice to excessive pollution and dehydrating agents: cigarette smoke, chemical fumes, alcohol, caffeine, dry air.
  Instead: − keep the air and your body clean and humid: drink 8−10 cups of non-caffeinated beverages daily, more if you exercise, drink alcohol or caffeine;
  − maintain 30% humidity in the air. Quit smoking!
- Don't slouch or adopt unbalanced postures.
  Instead: − learn and use good posture and alignment habits.

B.2 GRAVITY AND RELAXATION

You can take advantage of the force of gravity to help your muscles relax. Use the following exercises to learn about physical relaxation.

- Lying on the floor, give in to the force of gravity (Figure B.1). Notice which part of your body surrenders to gravity first, which part gives in next, and so on. Give each section permission to become heavier than it was when you first noticed it. If any parts of the body do not feel heavy once you have finished making rounds, concentrate on releasing these areas to the force of gravity. Allow your head to flop from side to side a few times, testing its weight. Notice the influence of gravity on your breathing. Take your time. Enjoy!

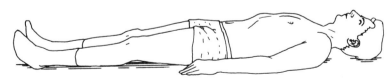

Figure B.1

- You can accomplish the same sense of relaxation sitting in the chair if you allow your body parts to succumb to gravity. Notice particularly the heaviness of your arms and legs, your chest, your face. You may drop your head forward on your chest to relax the neck. Now proceed with gravity exercises for the head.
- With your body upright, spine lengthened and neck free, tip the weight of your head slowly forward off the top of your neck, until you begin to feel gravity take over. After you reach the gravity threshold, roll your head back up on top of the neck and let it float freely. Test the threshold a few times this way, being sure to note the first sensation of weight transfer in the head. You should not need to move it more than a few centimetres to feel gravity taking over. Starting with your head balanced on top of the neck, drop it slowly backward, searching again for the first sign of weight transfer, and the force of gravity. Repeat. Use the same concept to define gravity boundaries on the sides of your head, by tipping the head slowly toward one ear, then the other. With practice and relaxation you should notice the gravity threshold moves closer to the center of your neck, and that the slightest movement of the head off the center in any direction makes you aware of its weight.

B.3 DYNAMIC ALIGNMENT: OPTIMIZING POSTURE FOR MOVEMENT

A healthy body posture is one where the skeletal system is properly aligned and the muscle system balanced. Such a system permits free movements throughout the body, without muscle strain. The movements that make up voice and speech involve specific muscles in the breathing system, larynx (voice box) and speech articulators. Misalignment of the body, or 'bad posture' can reduce freedom in speech movements at all levels.

The vocal system is best able to produce a wide range of pitches, intensities and qualities when the head, neck and back are well aligned so that no muscles are straining. Imagine a vertical line passing through the center of your back and neck to the crown of your head as though the spine were extended vertically. (If you're lying on your back while exploring this, the line will be a horizontal one.) Allow this image to 'lengthen' your whole body while it produces a natural structural line. This is a first approximation to body alignment. If all movements could be initiated from the crown of your head, then the rest of your body would fall into place below it, with the head, back and neck still aligned, the shoulders wide and low, the chest naturally expanded, and the limbs (arms and legs) resting or moving freely from the central structure. Your back also reaches its maximum width naturally with proper alignment, so the shoulder blades are flat, not pulled in toward each other. Your chest, back, and abdomen are now free to move as you breathe. The vertical 'release' of the spine frees the head from the neck at the base of the skull and permits it to move freely while still being 'lined up' with the spine.

Pointers: When the body is aligned, there should be no exaggerated 'hump' at the top of the back, the pelvis should be rocked backward slightly so the stomach is flat, and the lower back should have a slight concave shape. In vertical (standing or sitting) position your chin should be level, so there is approximately a $90°$ angle between the base of the jaw and the front of the neck. When you are standing, the knees should not be locked (Figure B.2a).

On the following pages, you will witness some examples of good and bad body alignment in various positions (Figure B.2b). Try to relate the concepts of alignment discussed above to each diagram, and decide which principles are being observed, or neglected, for each example. (Do these figures remind you of anyone you know?)

Here are some image-based exercises to practice 'lengthening' the spine; freeing the head, neck, shoulders, and back; and aligning the body:

1. Lie flat on your back and bend your knees up toward the ceiling. Place a 200–400-page book under the back of your head to reduce the curve in the back of your neck (the optimal book thickness depends on how far your head protrudes in the back: if your head is fairly flat in the back, this one may do nicely!). A firm pillow will also do, if it allows you to keep the neck straight, and release your head away from the neck. With your knees flexed, the curve in the lower back will be very small or non-existent (Figure B.2c).

   Now begin a lengthening process of your back and neck with your mind and body (let the mind be the leader). This should be a very gradual, gentle process. Increase the lengthening potential of your neck by freeing your head with a gentle side-to-side movement. Do not tilt your head back on your neck, rather let it lengthen and straighten. Let your back widen naturally against the floor. Make a mental note of the sensation of alignment and spine lengthening, to recreate it in standing and sitting positions.

2. Standing comfortably with your feet flat on the floor and knees unlocked, try to recreate the lengthened spine sensation you felt while lying down. Allow the crown of your head to be the highest point of your body and let it be drawn gently upward by some imaginary force. Let your neck lengthen without bending it, so it lengthens the spine along with it. Remember not to let your lower back collapse or tighten. Imagine your head is filled with helium gas and floating upward to the sky like a free balloon. Notice how your light head causes the spine to lengthen below it. Use very small horizontal movements to free the head from the neck and continue the lengthening process. Allow your shoulders to fall under the influence of gravity, so that they gain their maximum width. Imagine your spine is a column of upward-moving energy and allow it to support your body. To move forward, imagine you are being drawn gently upward and forward from the crown of the head, so that walking includes lengthening, and the head, neck, and back continue to be aligned. Let gravity influence the movements of your arms, legs, and breathing system (Figure B.2d).

3. Repeat (2) for sitting. Do not depend on furniture to align or support you, unless it can be adjusted to facilitate alignment. Use the sensations of your head floating freely above the neck, and spine lengthening to guide you in healthy sitting posture. To lean forward in the chair (such as you may do to eat, answer the phone, write . . .), allow the upper body to pivot freely from the hips and maintain the spine lengthening: don't thrust your body forward from your chin or chest! Remember, all movements are initiated from the crown of the head and involve lengthening the

POSTURE CHECKLIST

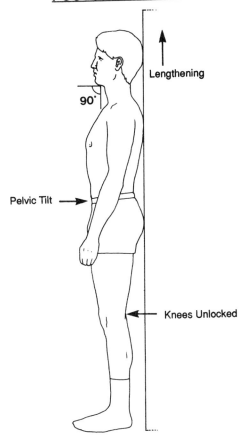

Lengthening

90°

Pelvic Tilt

Knees Unlocked

Figure B.2a

neck and back. Allow your shoulders to fall loosely on either side of the body so they reach maximum width. Use the loose head-shaking movements to free your head from your neck, allowing it to float above the body (Figure B.2e).

When you are sitting for extended periods, and working at a table, computer terminal, desk, etc., you should pull the chair in close to the table and arrange your work and monitor screen so you can keep your shoulders relaxed and your neck and back aligned. This takes a little ingenuity, but it is worthwhile!

4. To release muscle tension through your neck and back and increase lengthening potential, let the body hang forward, upside-down. From sitting posture, feet apart, pivot your upper body forward from the hips (lengthening as you do). Allow your head to drop forward onto your chest, of its own weight. The arms drop heavily to either side of the body. Now let the weight of your head and arms free the spine so it

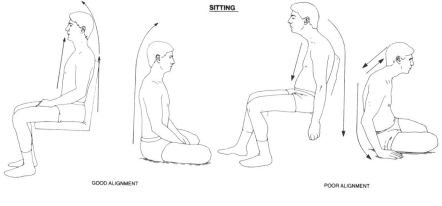

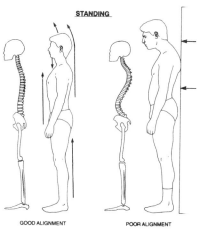

Figure B.2b

collapses forward from the top down. Hang forward loosely with your head and arms surrendering to gravity completely. As the back lengthens and widens allow the breath to move your back, widening the spaces in the lower back and between the shoulder blades. Shake your head loosely from side to side to loosen the neck muscles. Enjoy! Once you feel lengthened, or after a few minutes, begin slowly rebuilding the body structure from the bottom of your spine. Imagine each breath in inflates a small section of the body until it becomes vertical again. Continue the lengthening process, until only the head is hanging forward from its weight. Roll your head up the neck gradually and gently until the crown of the head is the highest part of the body again. Release the head upward off the neck, shaking it gently side to side. Feel taller? (Caution: if you have experienced any neck or back injury or feel any pain during the first part of this exercise, please do not continue. Consult your doctor and physical therapist before proceeding!)

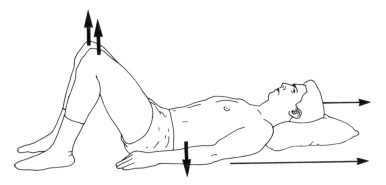

LYING SUPINE: LENGTHENING

Figure B.2c

5. Standing-to-sitting/sitting-to-standing: To maintain spine lengthening during this common daily activity, use the following principles. To stand from sitting position: with one foot placed ahead of the other, pivot forward from the hips; drop your head slightly forward, or release it upward and forward; relax your shoulders and arms; lengthen and roll forward into standing position. To sit from standing position: with one foot placed ahead of the other, drop your head and arms forward; lengthen and roll backward without tightening your lower back. Don't be afraid to use leg muscles to support the position change. (Figure B.2f).

Once your whole body is properly aligned, specific parts of the speech mechanism should be able to move freely. With your head, neck and back aligned and your head balanced lightly, your larynx, tongue, and jaw should be able to function more efficiently. Continue to practice good alignment in conjunction with specific exercises to free the voice and speech articulators.

B.4 SPECIFIC RELAXATION: LIBERATING THE SPEECH ARTICULATORS

B.4.1 Face

When the muscles of your face are free they allow your facial expressions to contribute to effective communication. On the other hand, if your face is constantly tense, it may distract people from what you say, and give the wrong impressions about your intent. Finally, if your face muscles are tense they can affect the quality and power of your voice by restricting movements of the speech articulators and resonators.

Here are some movements you should practice in front of a mirror if possible, to mobilize and relax your face muscles. Notice that some facial postures speak for themselves: for example, what meaning is conveyed by lowering/raising the eyebrows?

LENGTHENING AND WIDENING

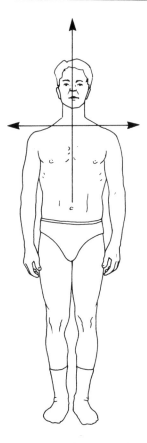

Figure B.2d

- Raise your eyebrows; hold; release. Lower your eyebrows; hold; release. Raise and lower your eyebrows repeatedly. Relax your eyebrows.
- Open your eyes very wide; hold; release. Squeeze your eyes closed tightly; hold; release. Open and close your eyes repeatedly. Relax your eyes.
- Squish your nose up; hold; release. Push your nose up and down repeatedly. Relax your nose.
- Push your cheeks up; hold; release. Push your cheeks up and down repeatedly. Relax your cheeks.
- Spread your lips wide across your face; hold; release. Push your lips forward to pucker them; hold; release. Spread and pucker your lips repeatedly. Relax your lips.
- Clench your jaw; hold; release. Flop your jaw up and down repeatedly. Relax your jaw.

LENGTHENING AND WIDENING

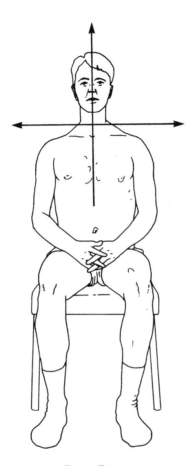

Figure B.2e

- Push your tongue against the roof of your mouth; hold; release. Let your tongue rest on the floor of your mouth; let your jaw drop open and breathe through your mouth.

Look for sensations of relaxation in the facial muscles: heaviness; warmth; tingling. Proceed with exercises to free the jaw, tongue, lips and throat.

B.4.2 Jaw

The jaw is a bone structure that is separate from the rest of the skeleton. However, it has muscle attachments to the cheekbones, the neck, the throat, the tongue, and the larynx.

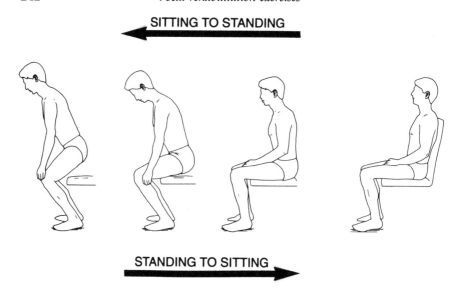

Figure B.2f

Tension in any of these muscles not only restricts the jaw during speech, but also reduces mobility in the areas attached to it. Many movements of the jaw are possible for biting, chewing, yawning, and facial expressions. One important type of movement dominates during relaxed speech. It is the simplest movement in many ways: a downward and backward rotation. The jaw drops down and slightly back to open, and rotates back up to close (Figure B.3). When the facial muscles are tense, the jaw may be very stiff or be pushed forward to open.

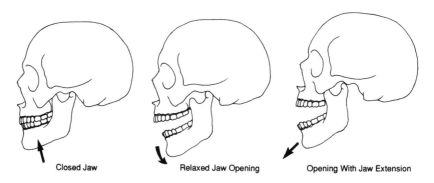

Figure B.3

The jaw joint is located directly in front of your ears. Place your fingers flat on top of the jaw joint while you open and close your jaw. Do you notice a bulging in the joint? This indicates the jaw is working too hard to open and close for speech. When the jaw is rotating simply without tension, there should be no obvious bulging in the sides of the face.

Grip your jaw firmly with your hand. Push it down and slightly back to open the jaw with the manual pressure. Don't try to open the jaw to its maximum width, only as far as your hand can coax it down. Do not help the movement with your face muscles! Your other hand can stay in front of your ear to make sure the jaw joint doesn't bulge. Push your open jaw closed with your hand, then let the jaw drop open again. Repeat this passive opening and closing motion until it feels free and easy. Make sure your tongue is not trying to participate in this activity: it should flat on the floor of the mouth and go along for the ride. Practice this exercise many times a day to reduce jaw tension and remind yourself of the passive jaw movement for speech. If you find your jaw is very tense and resistant, try an isometric exercise first:

clench your teeth together to tighten the jaw muscles; hold; release; repeat. Let the jaw relax open after the muscle work. Now close it again with your hand, and let it drop open afterward.

Sitting in a chair against a wall, drop your head back against the wall. Let your jaw fall away from your face to relax (take your time). Let your tongue relax on the floor of the mouth. Feel the force of gravity influencing your jaw position. Enjoy the heavy, relaxed sensation. With your hand, push your jaw closed, then take your hand away and let your jaw fall again. Enjoy the open throat feeling that comes with jaw relaxation. Let breath flow easily through your mouth.

The jaw movements we use in speech to articulate and resonate the sounds are simple, small and loose. They should be the same pivotal ones that your hand created. The jaw needs to be free of tension at all times so it can make very fast movements for speech articulation. It needs to be open during vowel sounds so they can resonate properly. Vowels are the longest sounds of speech so the jaw should be open or opening much of the time while we are speaking. In fact the jaw should never be closed tightly during speech.

You can feel the constant loose jaw movements during a simple syllable repetition. Try these sequences while watching your face in a mirror. You should see the jaw drop for each vowel. Make sure the movements are not confined to your lips or tongue!

Repeat these syllables at **normal speech speed**:

anananananananananananananan . . . (say the *a* vowels like *ah*).
Jaw starts from open position; jaw drops for each *a* vowel;

amamamamamamamamamamamamam . . .
Jaw starts from open position; jaw drops for each *a* vowel.

Try some other syllables. Allow gravity to do the work of opening the jaw for vowels. Make sure the jaw moves, not just the tongue or lips! Use a mirror:

ayaya. . .; asasa. . .; afafa. . .; alala. . .; apapa. . .; akaka. . .

Try some other vowels now. It feels more natural to open the jaw for 'open' vowels such as *a*; *ay*; *o* than for more 'closed' vowels such as *ee*; *oo*. Try to use the sensation of movement from the open vowels for all syllables:

> *onono. . .; arayray. . .; oosoosoo. . .; amama. . .; eemeemee. . .*

The principle movement of the jaw is still rotation down and back. This will feel awkward at first, but keeping gravity on your side will help. It may help to whisper the syllables first, then add your full voice.

Apply the same loose jaw movement to syllables that are speech. Start with series of words, such as counting, days of the week. Remember, the jaw drops for the vowel of each syllable. Use your regular speaking rate. Think of some speech phrases you use commonly and apply the loose-jaw principle to those. To keep the jaw in constant motion, imagine as you speak you are really saying something like: *ayayayaya. . .*

B.4.3 Tongue

Your tongue is really a big mass of muscles. It can make many different movements, including those we use for speech articulation. The back of the tongue is attached to the larynx (voice box). It also has attachments to the jaw, the palate and the throat. So when the tongue muscles are tense, they may not only make speech more effortful, but also make other parts of the throat, face, and neck tight. In its rest position, your tongue should lay flat on the floor of the mouth. You should feel it resting against the backs of the bottom teeth, including the molars. The back of the tongue should not be held high in the mouth or pulled back in the throat during rest or speech.

When the tongue base and jaw are both relaxed, you will be able to feel it in a simple way: the muscles under the chin, between the jaw bone and the front of the neck will be soft. Push your thumb into the fleshy area under your chin, as you see in the diagram (Figure B.4a). Release your jaw down and back by pushing with your forefinger, so you are breathing through your mouth. See how hollow and soft you can make the tongue and jaw muscles under your thumb. Now swallow, and notice the tension increase. This type of activity should not be felt during speech and singing.

Once you have the muscles relaxed, try prolonging some simple sounds: *aaaaaaaaaaah; ooooooooooh; aaaaaaaaaaay; hmmmmmmmmmmmmm; eeeeeeeeeeee*. Did you notice the tongue muscles tighten under your thumb during any of these sounds? You can use jaw and tongue relaxation, resonance and the coordinated voice onset to reduce this tension during speech.

Use the following exercise to learn about a forward, relaxed tongue position: Place your thumb under your chin to monitor tension. **Slowly** release your tongue forward over the bottom teeth and down, until it is stretched as far as possible. Let your jaw release down and back as the tongue releases forward. The muscles under your chin should stay soft. (If they tighten, you are **pushing** your tongue out instead of **releasing** it out.) Breathe through the big space that is created in your mouth while your tongue is stretching. Slowly relax the tongue back in the mouth, until it is resting low, flat and wide against the bottom teeth. Try vocalizing an easy *ah* now without any tongue movement.

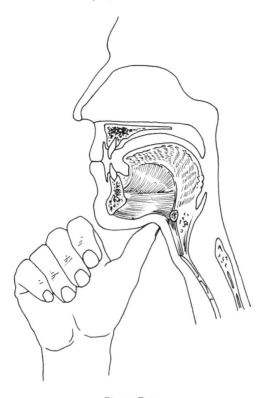

Figure B.4a

Use this exercise to release tension at the base of the tongue: With your hand, rotate your jaw open (down and back). Imagine the tip of your tongue is glued to the backs of your front bottom teeth (curl the tip of the tongue down under your bottom teeth). Once the tongue tip is fixed, release the back of your tongue forward, rolling gently like a wheel. Roll it all the way forward, then back in smooth, relaxed movements. Don't let your jaw or tongue tip move. Use a mirror to make sure the tongue is rolling forward. For a bigger stretch, curl the tongue under the teeth a little further. Your tongue should be spread wide as it comes forward, and should be free of bumps and grooves. (Figure B.4b)

Put a vocal sound behind the tongue rolling. You get: *hah Yah Yah Yah*. . . . The jaw should remain still.

Your tongue base should remain free of tension during speech, so that some of this rolling action is incorporated into articulation of sounds.

B.4.4 Lips

The lips are formed by a circular muscle: the 'puckering' muscle, that also lets you form speech sounds. If the face is tense, for example with a chronic tense social smile, the lips

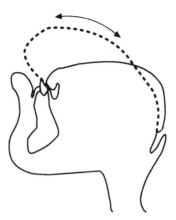

Figure B.4b

are not free to do their best job at speech articulation. When the upper lip is relaxed, the jaw can relax more easily.

Notice the feeling of a relaxed lower face when you whisper *oh*. The upper lip is stretched forward slightly, and the jaw drops.

Practice breathing through a big 'O' to stretch your lips and throat. Leave the tongue relaxed on the floor of your mouth. To release tension in the lip muscles, close them loosely, and blow air between them so they vibrate. See how long you can keep your lips vibrating on the airflow.

Here is an exercise to remind you what free lip movements feel like during speech: Start with the lips, jaw and tongue relaxed. Now gently whisper the sound sequence: *ooeeooeeooeeooee* . . ., with your lips moving freely forward for *oo* and stretching back for *ee*. Now try: *oayoayoayoayoay* . . . with your lips moving back and forth, not quite so far as for *ooee*, and your jaw relaxed open. Try the same sequences with full voice.

Many vowel and consonant sounds of speech should have forward lip movements. You should be aware of a constant activity in this area when you speak. Notice this particularly on the sounds: *oo; o; w; r; sh*.

B.4.5 Throat

By now you are aware that relaxation of the face, jaw, tongue and lips helps you achieve an 'open' relaxed throat sensation. Your throat should feel open while you vocalize for speech or singing. You can feel an exaggerated version of throat 'opening' during a yawn. Maintain that sensation after the yawn is finished.

With your jaw dropped, tongue and face relaxed, breathe through your mouth to relax your throat in preparation for speech or singing. To enhance the open throat feeling, drop your head back against the wall so your jaw drops low, and continue breathing through your mouth.

B.5 CO-ORDINATED VOICE ONSET

The onset of voice for speech or singing involves coordination of at least three actions:

- Release of breath from the lungs with activity in the muscles of the abdomen, chest and back;
- Approximation of the vocal folds so that the upward-flowing breath stream will set them into vibration;
- Resonance of the vocal tones, which may be felt as a 'buzzing' sensation in the various resonance cavities (mouth, face, sinuses, throat, chest)

You can experience naturally coordinated voice onset when you produce certain spontaneous vocal sounds. Laughing is one example of a co-ordinated voice onset. Another example is use of the expression *hm* instead of . . . Oh, that's interesting', or 'I get it', or 'I disagree'. During this vocal expression you can feel a co-ordinated voice onset, with the primary action in your abdomen. Your throat feels relaxed and 'open'. The same sensation may occur when you use *m hm* instead of 'yes', or 'I agree'. Try saying *hm* and *m hm* naturally, as if you really mean it. Notice where the principle muscle activity is. Don't attempt to plan or force this action: just observe how it occurs. Since both these expressions involve nasal resonance, you may feel a light buzzing sensation in your nose or face during the sound.

You can experience an **unco-ordinated** voice onset if you hold your breath before you make a sound. Try holding your breath while you say *ah*. Notice the 'klunk' at the beginning of the sound, and the feeling of throat effort and obstruction? This type of voice onset is wrong, and makes your throat feel tired because it is constantly resisting airflow from the lungs.

It is important for co-ordinated voice onset during speech that the structures in the breathing system are flexible and free of tension. You can test this by taking some short quick breaths in and out of your mouth, like a dog panting. Let the primary action originate in your abdomen, not high in the chest. You may also feel some breathing activity in your lower back. If you find tension in your body, return to relaxation and alignment exercises to free the breathing system before you proceed.

Co-ordinated voice onset is the fundamental mechanism for providing power during speech. You will feel the release of breath power most intensely if you start at a fairly low lung volume: that is, after you exhale excess air from the lungs. Sitting or lying quietly, observe the sensations of your body breathing. Notice the feelings associated with the end of the breath out, when your lungs are 'empty'. Prolong this low lung volume sensation for a few seconds, to become familiar with it. Feel the muscles getting ready to spring out and take a new breath in. Try *hm* after releasing most of the air out of your lungs, that is, at the 'empty' feeling. Be sure to let your abdomen relax after the sound, so more breath comes in, and you are ready to produce another sound: *hm*. Find a natural rhythm for repeating the coordinated voice onset, with respiratory release (RR) between sounds:

hm (RR) *hm* (RR) *hm* (RR) *hm* (RR) *hm* (RR) *hm* (RR) . . .

If you relax your chest and abdomen between sounds, you should find you can repeat the sound indefinitely at a rate of 2–4 times per second, without running out of air. This is possible because the RR is a respiratory release that actually lets you breathe in as much air as you used up for each *hm*. Since RR is a natural release after muscles contract, you should not have to think about breathing in between sounds: it occurs naturally when you relax the abdomen.

Use the same coordinated onset to make sounds with your mouth open. Drop your jaw and relax your tongue in the floor of your mouth. You may want to use a throat-relaxing position for this exercise: sitting in a chair against the wall, let your head lean heavily against the wall; allow your jaw to drop open and your tongue to relax in the floor of the mouth, so you find yourself breathing through your mouth. Release the sound: *huh* without moving your tongue, jaw, lips, or face. The sound *huh* has the same potential meanings as *hm*: 'Oh, that's interesting', or 'I get it', or 'I disagree'. Think about the meaning behind the sound.

If you feel effort in your throat or face when you start sounds, you should reduce it by monitoring your tongue muscles under your chin (section 13.4.3). If your tongue is really stubborn about helping the sound start, wrap some gauze cloth around it and hold it out firmly with your hand while you learn how to make the sounds without tongue action.

Once you feel comfortable with rhythmic repeated onsets for *hm* and *huh*, experiment with sound extension. All you need to do is hold on to the sound energy a little longer each time, keeping the abdominal muscles engaged to give the sound continued power.
So you have:

   hm (RR) *hmm* (RR) *hmmmm* (RR) *hmmmmmmm* . . .

or:

   huh (RR) *huuh* (RR) *huuuuh* (RR) *huuuuuuh* . . .

Try sustaining the sounds as long as possible: until your abdomen is unable to squeeze any more air out. Let the respiratory release (RR) occur naturally afterwards so you are ready to sustain another sound. It is very important not to try and direct the breath in even for very long or loud sounds: just let the voice onset muscles relax and the breath will come in naturally. This way you will not 'overstuff' the lungs with air, by tensing muscles of the upper chest and neck. Notice as you sustain sounds longer and use more breath energy to do so, the body responds by taking more breath in, to prepare for the next voice onset. During speech, you should not keep talking until you are completely 'empty' of air, like you just did for sustained sounds, but using the air at the bottom of the breath tank in this exercise will help acquaint you with the voice-sustaining muscles. Once you can sustain sounds comfortably, using the lower breathing muscles to keep energy flowing, try increasing the loudness of sounds toward the end. Let the abdominal muscles take the responsibility for increasing loudness on: *huuuuuuuuuuuuuuuuh*.

Can you imagine each sustained sound is actually a sentence? Try 'thinking' speech sentences while you are extending coordinated voice onsets of various lengths.

You should be able to add some movements of the speech articulators to the extended vocal sounds now so the sounds resemble repeated syllables. Start with coordinated voice onsets, then let the tongue, jaw or lips move throughout the sound so you have a speech-like sound sequence:

> *hunununuh* . . .; *hulululuh* . . .; *humumumu* . . .; *huwuwuwu* . . .

You can produce all the vowels and vowel-like sounds in speech with a coordinated voice onset. Use a soft *h* to make sure the initiating action begins with the breathing system. Try different vowel shapes in your mouth, with the coordinated voice onset. You should monitor the tongue muscles under your chin with your thumb to be sure you don't use any throat tension to start sounds (section 13.4.3).

Here we go:

> *hey* (RR) *hey* (RR) *hey* (RR) *hey* . . .
> *hee* (RR) *hee* (RR) *hee* (RR) *hee* . . .
> *ho* (RR) *ho* (RR) *ho* (RR) *ho* . . .
> *hoo* (RR) *hoo* (RR) *hoo* (RR) *hoo* . . .
> *hi* (RR) *hi* (RR) *hi* (RR) *hi* . . .
> *hr* (RR) *hr* (RR) *hr* (RR) *hr* . . .

Say some words using the coordinated voice onset: . . . Hey! Hi! 'Really?' 'No!' 'No way!' 'Fine' 'Sure' 'OK' 'For sure!' . . .

Since you already know how to extend the coordinated voice onset, using it for speech is simply a matter of maintaining a relaxed throat, initiating the sound correctly, and using abdominal muscles to keep the energy flowing from the breathing center. Don't forget to release the respiratory muscles (RR) between sentences!

Say:

> 'Hey there, Mary' (RR) 'How's it going?'

Think:

> (*huuuuuuuuuuuuuh* (RR) *huuuuuuuuuuuuuh?*)

> 'Will you please open the window?' (RR) 'Thanks!'
> (*huuuuuuuuuuuuuuuuuuuuuuuuuuuuuh?* (RR) *huh!*)

> 'No way I can have that order ready by Monday, (RR) sir!'
> (*huuuuuuuuuuuuuuuuuuuuuuuuuuuuuuuuuuuuuuuuuuuuuh,* (RR) *huh!*)

(Note: a comma (,) means (RR) if you're out of breath energy)

Getting the idea? Good!

B.6 FEEDING THE RESONATORS AND MMMMAKING THE MMMMOST OF RESONANCE

Acoustic resonance means amplification of the voice. You can feel resonance in your vocal tract when it is open, and sufficient sound energy is being supplied to 'feed' the resonators. Explore the sensation of vocal resonance using nasal sounds first:

> *hmmmmmmmmmmmmmmmmmm*; *hnnnnnnnnnnnnnnnn*; *hngngngngngngngngn*

(*hng* is the sound at the end of 'sing').

You will, of course, use a coordinated voice on set to initiate these resonating sounds.

Where do you feel a resonance ('buzzing') sensation? lips? nose? head? throat? palate? teeth? chest?

Continue to experiment with nasal resonators in conjunction with an open throat, coordinated voice onset, and different positions:

- hum lying on your back
- hum hanging forward from the hips, either standing or sitting
- hum with your head dropped forward/back

Experiment with different pitches and gradual pitch changes during the hum. Does the buzzing change location or intensity with pitch changes? Remember to keep your jaw and tongue passive when you are changing pitches.

Your tongue muscles under your chin should stay passive while you are humming. Check them with your thumb. (section B.4.3)

You can extend the buzzing sensation from humming into non-nasal sounds. Try saying some words loaded with nasal sounds, and lift and extend the buzz right through the vowel sounds. Make sure your jaw drops open for the vowels!:

Mmmmmmaaaaaaaannnnnnn (man)
Mmmmmmiiiiiiiinnnnnnn (mine)
Mmmmmmaaaaaaaannnnnnnnyyyyyyy (many)
Nnnnnniiiiiiiinnnnnnn (nine)
Nnnnnnaaaaaaaammmmmmmm (name)
Nnnnnnaaaaaaaammmmmmmmmiiiiiiiingngngngng (naming)

Don't let the pitch or energy drop low toward the ends of words so they rattle in your throat: keep them buzzing throughout!

Try combining several words into phrases, so you have continuous resonance sensation in speech. Continue to prolong the nasal and vowel sounds so they buzz:

Mmmmmmmmmooooooorrrmmmmmoooooonnnneeeey (more money)
Mmmmyyyynnnaaaammmmiiiismmmaaaaryyyyy. (My name is Mary.)
Nnnniiiciyyyeeennnuuunnnciiiaaatd! (Nicely enunciated!)

(Think up some more sentences with lots of nasal buzz)

Other sounds can buzz too!

You probably noticed during the last humming exercise that many sounds have resonance sensations. Since vowels are naturally the loudest speech sounds, they have the greatest potential for resonance power. This is convenient, since vowels make up the longest segments of speech. Powerful vowels means powerful speech.

As with humming, all that is required to achieve good vowel resonance is an open vocal tract and continuous voice energy from your breathing center. The vocal sound will find its way to the resonating cavities as long as these conditions are met. Prepare your vocal tract first:

- sitting in a chair drop your head back against the wall;
- drop your jaw open;
- make sure your tongue is passive;
- stretch the upper lip down to form O.

Using a coordinated voice onset, initiate and sustain the vowel:

'hooooooooooooooooooooo. . ..' (keep your throat open!)

Where do you feel a resonance sensation? palate? head? throat? chest? lips? teeth? sinuses? elsewhere?

Try some other vowel shapes:

'hoo oo oo oo oo oo oo oo oo. . .' (lips further forward)

'hee ee ee ee ee ee ee ee ee. . .' (maintain a bit of lip rounding, but let the tongue roll forward from its base.

'haaaaaaaaaaaaaaaaaaaaaaaaaaaa. . .' (tongue flat, jaw slack)

Each vowel has its own resonance characteristic and sensation. Let each one find its maximum potential for power, by keeping the resonators open. Try some different positions: lying on your back; head dropped forward. If you have trouble keeping the jaw passively open for the resonance exercise, you can prop a thin slice of cork between your molars, so you're holding it gently between your teeth on the round edge. Let your upper lip stretch over your top teeth gently, so the resonance sensation comes 'forward' to the lips.

Since you already know how to move the jaw passively for syllable repetitions, you can combine these movements with vowel resonance exercises.

'hamamamamama. . .'; 'hononononono. . .'; 'heyeyeyeyey. . .'

(Section B.4.2 has more syllable combinations, or make some up)

Now you can use natural speech movements to enhance continuous resonance sensations. Start with word series: counting, days. . . Let the resonance flow from one vowel to the next in each phrase.

B.7 EXTENDING YOUR DYNAMIC PITCH RANGE

One of the most remarkable things about the human voice is its potential to create a wide range of different pitches. Your usual speaking pitches reflect only part of the full range your voice is capable of making. Certain special sound effects can help you increase your vocal flexibility and quality. Use the following exercises to achieve your maximum potential dynamic pitch range for speaking and singing.

B.7.1 Bubbling and Trilling

Your lips can vibrate in much the same way your vocal folds do when air flows between them. Press your upper and lower lips together lightly. Keeping them together, blow air between your lips, so you get: *pbrbrbrbrbrbrbr* . . . (turn your vocal motor on). Extend this tone as long as you can, using the power from your breathing system to keep it going. Once you have mastered the sound extension, start it at a higher pitch and let it slowly glide down. Make sure the sound begins with lip bubbling, and that your lips continue to vibrate throughout the whole sound. This ensures you are supporting the sound with air flow energy, and not tensing your mouth and throat. Start a little higher each time, using the lip-bubble as the primary effect. Try gliding up and down in pitch. Notice how much work the breathing system has to do to keep it going! Your throat, tongue and jaw should remain passive and relaxed. Monitor the tongue muscles under your chin to be sure they remain passive (section B.4.3).

If lip bubbling is difficult for you, you can use a tongue trill to extend your pitch range. This sound is made by allowing your tongue tip to vibrate against the roof of your mouth, like rolling the r sound. Start it like this: *tdrdrdrdrdrdrdr* . . . (turn on your vocal motor so you hear the tone). Keep your throat, jaw, and tongue passive, and let the airflow do the work of maintaining the trill. Monitor your tongue base muscles under your chin to make certain you don't tighten your tongue and throat. Once you have mastered the sound extension, start it at higher pitches and let it slowly glide down. Make sure the sound starts with tongue trilling each time, and continue trilling throughout the sound, to keep your mouth and throat relaxed. Try gliding up and down on the trill to explore your dynamic pitch range. Notice the sensations of passive jaw, tongue and throat while you are vocalizing throughout your range.

B.7.2. Vocal Siren

The human voice is capable of producing sounds that are so clear they resemble sirens. Before you explore your vocal siren, use your finger to ensure a constant flow of air will support the sound. Place your index finger vertically on your lips in the gesture you use to say *sh* . . . (that is to quiet or 'shush' people) (Figure B.5). With your throat open, jaw and tongue passive and lips forward, extend the sound *oo* so it buzzes on your finger. You should hear a secondary sound as the airflow contacts your finger, like the sound a kazoo makes. Notice it takes respiratory effort to maintain this secondary vibration. Glide up and down in pitch while maintaining the *oo* and secondary vibration. Can you feel the *oo* sound resonating anywhere?

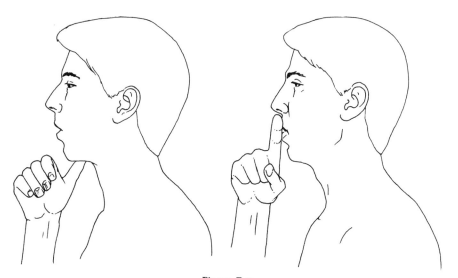

Figure B.5

Now try the vocal siren without monitoring the finger-buzz. Use a relaxed *oo* which starts with a coordinated voice onset. Feel and listen to the sound as it glides gently up and down in pitch like a siren. Let the siren achieve its maximum resonance sensation in your mouth, sinus and facial cavities. Keep your throat open, and jaw and tongue passive (use your thumb under your chin to monitor the base of tongue muscles)

Start the sounds light and high on *hoo* . . . and let them glide gently down. Notice any changes in resonance sensation as you glide down. Remember that continuous and steady airflow contributes to a clear siren at all pitches, so the breathing center must stay involved throughout this exercise.

The siren effect can be created on any vocal sounds that 'buzz'. Try the siren on sounds you found particularly resonant during previous exercises: *mmm* . . ., *nnn* . . .; *ngngng* . . .; *eeeeee* . . .; *rrr* . . .; *aaa.* . .. Make sure muscles of your face and throat don't try to participate in this effect! Look for the same vibrant resonance sensations on soft and louder sirens. The pitch-changing effort should come from your breathing muscles, not your throat!

Index

Page numbers in italics refer to Figures.